Medical Librarian 2.0: Use of Web 2.0 Technologies in Reference Services

M. Sandra Wood, MLS, MBA, AHIP, FMLA
Editor

Medical Librarian 2.0: Use of Web 2.0 Technologies in Reference Services has been co-published simultaneously as *Medical Reference Services Quarterly*, Volume 26, Supplement #1 2007.

Medical Librarian 2.0:
Use of Web 2.0 Technologies
in Reference Services

Medical Librarian 2.0:Use of Web 2.0 Technologies in Reference Services has been co-published simultaneously as *Medical Reference Services Quarterly*, Volume 26, Supplement #1 2007.

The Haworth Information Press®
An Imprint of The Haworth Press, Inc.

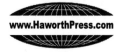

www.HaworthPress.com

Medical Librarian 2.0:Use of Web 2.0 Technologies in Reference Services has been co-published simultaneously as *Medical Reference Services Quarterly*™, Volume 26, Supplement #1 2007.

The development, preparation, and publication of this work has been undertaken with great care. However, the publisher, employees, editors, and agents of The Haworth Press and all imprints of The Haworth Press, Inc., including The Haworth Medical Press® and Pharmaceutical Products Press®, are not responsible for any errors contained herein or for consequences that may ensue from use of materials or information contained in this work. With regard to case studies, identities and circumstances of individuals discussed herein have been changed to protect confidentiality. Any resemblance to actual persons, living or dead, is entirely coincidental.

The Haworth Press is committed to the dissemination of ideas and information according to the highest standards of intellectual freedom and the free exchange of ideas. Statements made and opinions expressed in this publication do not necessarily reflect the views of the Publisher, Directors, management, or staff of The Haworth Press, Inc., or an endorsement by them.

Library of Congress Cataloging-in-Publication Data

Medical librarian 2.0 : Use of Web 2.0 Technologies in Reference Services / M. Sandra Wood, editor.
p. cm.
"Co-published simultaneously as Medical references services quarterly, volume 26, supplement #1 2007."
Includes bibliographical references and index.
ISBN-13: 978-0-7890-3605-6 (alk. paper)
ISBN-13: 978-0-7890-3606-3 (pbk. : alk. paper)
1. Medical libraries–Reference services. 2. Internet in library reference services. 3. Medical libraries–Information technology. I. Wood, M. Sandra. II. Medical reference services quarterly.
Z675.M4M37 2007
025.5'27661–dc22

2007033829

The HAWORTH PRESS Inc.
Abstracting, Indexing & Outward Linking
PRINT and ELECTRONIC BOOKS & JOURNALS

This section provides you with a list of major indexing & abstracting services and other tools for bibliographic access. That is to say, each service began covering this periodical during the year noted in the right column. Most Websites which are listed below have indicated that they will either post, disseminate, compile, archive, cite or alert their own Website users with research-based content from this work. (This list is as current as the copyright date of this publication.)

Abstracting, Website/Indexing Coverage . . . . Year When Coverage Began

- **(IBR) International Bibliography of Book Reviews on the Humanities and Social Sciences (Thomson)**
  <http://www.saur.de> · 2006

- **(IBZ) International Bibliography of Periodical Literature on the Humanities and Social Sciences (Thomson)**
  <http://www.saur.de> · 2004

- ****Academic Search Premier (EBSCO)****
  <http://www.epnet.com/academic/acasearchprem.asp> · · · · · · 2004

- ****Biological Abstracts (Thomson Scientific)****
  <http://www.biosis.org> · 1983

- ****BIOSIS PREVIEWS (Thomson Scientific)**** · · · · · · · · · · · · · · 1983

- ****BIOSIS Selective Coverage Unique (Thomson Scientific)**** · · · · 2006

- ****CINAHL (Cumulative Index to Nursing & Allied Health Literature) (EBSCO)**** <http://www.cinahl.com> · · · · · · · · · · 1982

- ****CINAHL Plus (EBSCO)**** · 2006

- ****INSPEC (The Institution of Engineering and Technology)****
  <http://www.iee.org.uk/publish/> · · · · · · · · · · · · · · · · · · · 1983

- ****LISA: Library and Information Science Abstracts (Cambridge Scientific Abstracts)****
  <http://www.csa.com/factsheets/list-set-c.php> · · · · · · · · · · · · 1989

- ****MasterFILE Premier (EBSCO)****
  <http://www.epnet.com/government/mfpremier.asp> · · · · · · · · · 2006

(continued)

- ****MEDLINE (National Library of Medicine)****
  <http://www.nlm.nih.gov> ·································· 1984
- ****PubMed** <http://www.ncbi.nlm.nih.gov/pubmed/>** ········ 1984
- *Academic Search Alumni Edition (EBSCO)*
  <http://www.epnet.com>································· 2007
- *Academic Search Complete (EBSCO)* ······················ 2007
- *Academic Source Premier (EBSCO)* ······················· 2007
- *Biomeditaties (Biomedical Information of the Dutch Library*
  Association) <http://www.nvb-online.nl> ················ 2003
- *British Library Inside (The British Library)*
  <http://www.bl.uk/services/current/inside.html>············ 2006
- *Cabell's Directory of Publishing Opportunities in Educational*
  Technology & Library Science <http://www.cabells.com>····· 2006
- *Cambridge Scientific Abstracts <http://www.csa.com>* ········· 2006
- *Chartered Institute of Library and Information Professionals*
  (CILIP) Health Libraries Newsletter "Current Literature"
  (Published quarterly by Blackwell Science.)
  <http://www.blackwell-science.com/hlr/newsletter/> ········ 1999
- *Consumer Health Complete (EBSCO)* ···················· 2006
- *DH-Data (available via DataStar and in the HMIC*
  [Health Management Information Consortium] CD ROM)···· 2004
- *EBSCOhost Electronic Journals Service (EJS)*
  <http://ejournals.ebsco.com>···························· 2001
- *Electronic Collections Online (OCLC)*
  <http://www.oclc.org/electroniccollections/> ·············· 2006
- *Elsevier Eflow-l* ······································· 2006
- *Elsevier Scopus <http://www.info.scopus.com>* ·············· 2003
- *EMCare(Elsevier) <http://www.elsevier.com>*················ 2006
- *European Association for Health Information & Libraries:*
  Selected abstracts in newsletter "Publications" section ······ 1995
- *Google <http://www.google.com>*·························· 2004
- *Google Scholar <http://scholar.google.com>* ··············· 2004
- *Haworth Document Delivery Center*
  <http://www.HaworthPress.com/journals/dds.asp> ·········· 1982
- *Health Source: Nursing/Academic Edition (EBSCO)*
  <http://www.epnet.com/academic/hsnursing.asp> ··········· 2006

(continued)

(continued)

- *SwetsWise* <http://www.swets.com> · **2001**
- *TOC Premier (EBSCO)*· **2007**
- *WilsonWeb* <http://vnweb.hwwilsonweb.com/hww/Journals/>· · · · **2005**
- *zetoc (The British Library)* <http://www.bl.uk>· · · · · · · · · · · · · · · **2004**

Bibliographic Access

- **Cabell's Directory of Publishing Opportunities in Educational Curriculum and Methods <http://www.cabells.com/>**
- **Magazines for Libraries (Katz)**
- **MediaFinder <http://www.mediafinder.com/>**
- **Ulrich's Periodicals Directory: The Global Source for Periodicals Information Since 1932 <http://www. bowkerlink.com>**

The following services provide select coverage of Medical Reference Services Quarterly *abstracts and articles:*

Computer & Control Abstracts (INSPEC)
Electrical & Electronics Abstracts (INSPEC)
Physics Abstracts (INSPEC)

Special Bibliographic Notes related to special journal issues (separates) and indexing/abstracting:

- indexing/abstracting services in this list will also cover material in any "separate" that is co-published simultaneously with Haworth's special thematic journal issue or DocuSerial. Indexing/abstracting usually covers material at the article/chapter level.
- monographic co-editions are intended for either non-subscribers or libraries which intend to purchase a second copy for their circulating collections.
- monographic co-editions are reported to all jobbers/wholesalers/approval plans. The source journal is listed as the "series" to assist the prevention of duplicate purchasing in the same manner utilized for books-in-series.
- to facilitate user/access services all indexing/abstracting services are encouraged to utilize the co-indexing entry note indicated at the bottom of the first page of each article/chapter/contribution.
- this is intended to assist a library user of any reference tool (whether print, electronic, online, or CD-ROM) to locate the monographic version if the library has purchased this version but not a subscription to the source journal.
- individual articles/chapters in any Haworth publication are also available through the Haworth Document Delivery Service (HDDS).

As part of
Haworth's
continuing
commitment
to better serve
our library
patrons,
we are
proud to
be working
with the
following
electronic
services:

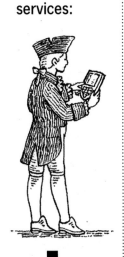

AGGREGATOR SERVICES

EBSCOhost

Ingenta

J-Gate

Minerva

OCLC FirstSearch

Oxmill

SwetsWise

LINK RESOLVER SERVICES

1Cate (Openly Informatics)

ChemPort
(American Chemical Society)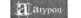

CrossRef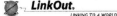

Gold Rush (Coalliance)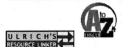

LinkOut (PubMed)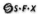

LINKplus (Atypon)

LinkSolver (Ovid)

LinkSource with A-to-Z (EBSCO)

Resource Linker (Ulrich)

SerialsSolutions (ProQuest)

SFX (Ex Libris)

Sirsi Resolver (SirsiDynix)

Tour (TDnet)

Vlink (Extensity, formerly Geac)

WebBridge (Innovative Interfaces)

Medical Librarian 2.0: Use of Web 2.0 Technologies in Reference Services

CONTENTS

ABOUT THE EDITOR

M. Sandra Wood, MLS, MBA, AHIP, FMLA, is Librarian Emerita, Pennsylvania State University. Previously, she was Librarian, Reference and Database Services, The George T. Harrell Library, The Milton S. Hershey Medical Center, The Pennsylvania State University College of Medicine, Hershey, PA. She has over 35 years of experience as a medical reference librarian, with experience/interests in general reference, management of reference services, database and Internet searching , and user instruction. Ms. Wood has been widely published in the field of medical reference and is Editor of *Medical Reference Services Quarterly, Journal of Consumer Health on the Internet*, and Co-editor of the *Journal of Electronic Resources in Medical Libraries* (Haworth). She is author of the Haworth book, *Internet Guide to Cosmetic Surgery for Women*, published in 2005, and *Internet Guide to Cosmetic Surgery for Men*, published in 2006, and is editor or co-editor of several other Haworth books, including *Women's Health on the Internet, Health Care Resources on the Internet: A Guide for Librarians and Health Care Consumers, Men's Health on the Internet*, and *Cancer Resources on the Internet*. She is a member of the Medical Library Association and the Special Libraries Association, and has served on the MLA's Board of Directors as Treasurer. Ms. Wood is also a Fellow of the Medical Library Association.

Medical Librarian 2.0:
Use of Web 2.0 Technologies
in Reference Services

M. Sandra Wood

INTRODUCTION

In less than a decade, the Internet has become a routine part of most people's lives. What is truly amazing, though, is how this service has revolutionized almost everything that we do, from sending mail (e-mail versus snail mail) to banking, shopping, meeting and making friends, and more. Long-term Internet users have seen the move from text-based interfaces to GUIs (graphical user interfaces), from Gophers to Web sites, from the original Internet to the World Wide Web.

Librarians have been at the forefront in using the Web. Once the potential of the Web was recognized, electronic services such as the online catalog and electronic databases were moved quickly from local and CD-ROM based services to online availability via the Internet. Libraries developed their own Web sites, creating links to heavily used resources to facilitate easy access for their users. By the start of the new millennium, just about everyone had a Web site; governments, associations, academic institutions, corporations, and more, had realized that they could provide information via the Internet for users/consumers to read. It was a one-way street, from provider to consumer. However, by the late 1990s, social networking sites were springing up on the Web.

[Haworth co-indexing entry note]: "Medical Librarian 2.0: Use of Web 2.0 Technologies in Reference Services." Wood, M. Sandra. Co-published simultaneously in *Medical Reference Services Quarterly* (The Haworth Information Press, an imprint of The Haworth Press, Inc.) Vol. 26, Supp. #1, 2007, pp. 1-3; and: *Medical Librarian 2.0: Use of Web 2.0 Technologies in Reference Services* (ed: M. Sandra Wood) The Haworth Information Press, an imprint of The Haworth Press, Inc., 2007, pp. 1-3. Single or multiple copies of this article are available for a fee from The Haworth Document Delivery Service [1-800-HAWORTH, 9:00 a.m. - 5:00 p.m. (EST). E-mail address: docdelivery@haworthpress.com].

These sites were not static, but were user-driven. They offered interactive, user-focused capabilities that were quickly adopted by the general public. Where previously, content was posted on a Web site and only authorized persons could change the content, the "new" Web allowed, even encouraged, input from the user. Now called Web 2.0, these new technologies encourage interaction between Internet users–social networking–and a whole new vocabulary has sprung up: tagging, cloud tags, folksonomies, RSS, blogs, syndication, podcasting, streaming video, wikis, wikipedia, MySpace, social software, mashups, instant messaging, chat. This list could go on and on. Librarians have recognized the potential of Web 2.0 technologies and are moving quickly to adapt and use these tools for reference and user services.

This monographic supplement to *Medical Reference Services Quarterly* brings together a group of original papers about the use of Web 2.0 technologies for the provision of reference services. The focus is on health sciences libraries, but the concepts are applicable to all types of libraries; in fact, some of the technologies have been better adapted in public and general academic libraries. By the time this volume is published, newer technologies will have appeared, as the Web is constantly changing. The technologies described here, though, show great promise for use by libraries in their constant search to be more relevant to their users.

Elizabeth Connor begins the volume with an overview of Library 2.0, focusing on Web 2.0 technologies as used by libraries. She defines and describes the technologies and discusses planning for future library services along with implications of teaching users who were "born digital."

The second paper is a review of "Virtual Reference Services in Academic Health Sciences Libraries," by Ana D. Cleveland and Jodi L. Philbrick. After reviewing virtual reference services and discussing key issues, they describe their study of virtual reference in academic health sciences libraries in the United States and Canada. Virtual reference is truly one of the initial Internet 2.0 services used by libraries. Initially, libraries purchased special software to provide this service, but as chat and instant messaging have become more prevalent, these technologies are being utilized by libraries to provide virtual reference.

Alexia D. Estabrook and David L. Rothman describe RSS (really simple syndication), which is being used for blogs, databases, and other Web-based sources. One major use is for selective dissemination of information, opening a way automatically to push selected information to patrons.

Nadine Ellero, Ryan Looney, and Bart Ragon describe podcasting, calling it a "disruptive technology." They discuss the technology in general and then give specific examples of how it has been used by librarians, and taught to users, at the Claude Moore Health Sciences Library. The specific issue of cataloging this medium is described.

In "Streams of Consciousness: Streaming Video in Health Sciences Libraries," Nancy T. Lombardo, Sharon E. Dennis, and Derek Cowan review the history of streaming media on the Web, along with library uses of this technology. They describe the use of streaming and on-demand video services provided by the Spencer S. Eccles Health Sciences Library, a library which has been a leader in the use of this technology.

Melissa L. Rethlefsen introduces the reader to the concept of social networking, and to social networking tools such as MySpace, Facebook, and Vox. Specific library-related tools include LibraryThing, Flickr, and del.icio.us, and Rethlefsen describes how these technologies can be useful to all types of libraries.

In "Content Management and Web 2.0 with Drupal," Chad M. Fennell describes the University of Minnesota Health Sciences Libraries' selection and use of Drupal as a content management tool. The specifics for local installation are detailed for this open source software.

In "It's a Wiki Wiki World," Mary Carmen Chimato introduces wikis, which can be used both internally for sharing information among library staff, and externally, for communicating with library users. She describes some unique and interesting uses for this social software tool, ranging from an institutional repository to an online journal club.

Mashups blend two or more programs to produce a new, enhanced program. In "Mashing Up the Internet," Michelle A. Kraft, well known for her Krafty Librarian blog, describes how mashups can be used in medical libraries, and also raises some concerns about data and security.

Many librarians, especially those new to the field who have grown up with computers, have been quick to adopt Web 2.0 technologies. Other librarians may be just beginning to look at how these tools will impact their ability to provide new services. Whether you are a current user of Web 2.0 tools, or the concepts are new to you, this volume will provide a good foundation about the most popular Web 2.0/Library 2.0 technologies at the time the papers were written (late 2006), and will introduce librarians to the terminology, some existing uses of the technologies, and potential uses of these tools. To remain relevant to their users, libraries must provide services that users want and will use; Web 2.0 technologies facilitate libraries getting the right information to the right user at the right time. Hopefully, the creative examples of ways to use new technologies, as described in this volume, will stimulate readers to adapt and adopt Web 2.0 technologies in their libraries, to provide new services that will benefit both the libraries and their users.

Library 2.0: An Overview

Elizabeth Connor

SUMMARY. Web 2.0 technologies focus on peer production, posting, subscribing, and tagging content; building and inhabiting social networks; and combining existing and emerging applications in new and creative ways to impart meaning, improve search precision, and better represent data. The Web 2.0 extended to libraries has been called Library 2.0, which has ramifications for how librarians, including those who work in medical settings, will interact and relate to persons who were born digital, especially related to teaching and learning, and planning future library services and facilities. doi:10.1300/J115v26S01_02 *[Article copies available for a fee from The Haworth Document Delivery Service: 1-800-HAWORTH. E-mail address: <docdelivery@haworthpress.com> Website: <http://www. HaworthPress.com> © 2007 by The Haworth Press, Inc. All rights reserved.]*

KEYWORDS. Web 2.0, read/write Web, Library as Place, Library 2.0, Librarian 2.0, Medical Library 2.0, Medical Librarian 2.0, Semantic Web, Web 3.0, blogs, mashups, podcasting, wikis, blikis, folksonomy, tagging, tag clouds, peer production, user-generated content, syndication, social networking, forecasting, future trends, medical libraries, medical education

Elizabeth Connor, MLS, AHIP (elizabeth.connor@citadel.edu) is Science Liaison and Associate Professor of Library Science, Daniel Library, The Citadel, the Military College of South Carolina, 171 Moultrie Street, Charleston, SC 29409-6140.

[Haworth co-indexing entry note]: "Library 2.0: An Overview." Connor, Elizabeth. Co-published simultaneously in *Medical Reference Services Quarterly* (The Haworth Information Press, an imprint of The Haworth Press, Inc.) Vol. 26, Supp. #1, 2007, pp. 5-23; and: *Medical Librarian 2.0: Use of Web 2.0 Technologies in Reference Services* (ed: M. Sandra Wood) The Haworth Information Press, an imprint of The Haworth Press, Inc., 2007, pp. 5-23. Single or multiple copies of this article are available for a fee from The Haworth Document Delivery Service [1-800-HAWORTH, 9:00 a.m. - 5:00 p.m. (EST). E-mail address: docdelivery@haworthpress.com].

INTRODUCTION

Web 2.0 technologies have the potential to transform medical library practice in ways more profound than the changes caused by the first-generation Internet. Widespread acceptance and use of the World Wide Web in the office and at home have eclipsed many other technological advances. Brown likens the transformative nature of the Web to the technological and cultural breakthroughs caused by the invention of the first electric generator, and the subsequent infrastructure developed to support that invention.[1] Because many of the next-generation tools associated with Web 2.0 are already in existence and common use, the significance of Web 2.0 as a call to action may have gone unnoticed or been dismissed as hyperbole by some experienced librarians, especially in medical settings. The extension of Web 2.0 principles to librarianship has been dubbed Library 2.0 or Librarian 2.0. Much of the literature on the subject of Library 2.0 involves public libraries or university libraries, and can be found in blog postings or mainstream library publications such as *American Libraries*, *Library Journal*, and *Computers in Libraries*. Tim O'Reilly's original musings on the subject are worthwhile reading.[2]

Blogger librarian Sarah Houghton defines the trend in this way:

> Library 2.0 simply means making your library space (virtual and physical) more interactive, collaborative, and driven by community needs. Examples of where to start include blogs, gaming nights for teens, and collaborative photo sites. The basic drive is to get people back into the library by making the library relevant to what they want and need in their daily lives . . . to make the library a destination and not an afterthought.[3]

Understanding of Library 2.0 as a concept rather than a meaningless buzzword has been further confounded by the lack of consensus on the subject. Meredith Farkus defines it in terms of library operations:

> The idea of Library 2.0 represents a significant paradigm shift in the way we view library services. It's about a seamless user experience, where usability, interoperability, and flexibility of library systems is key. It's about the library being more present in the community through programming, community building (both online and physical), and outreach via technology (IM, screencasting, blogs, wikis, etc.). It's about allowing user participation through writing reviews

and tagging in the catalog and making their voice heard through blogs and wikis. It's about making the library more transparent through its Web presence and its physical design. We need to make the library human, ubiquitous, and user-centered. This involves a change in our systems, our Web presence, and our very attitudes. It will take a lot of work for a library to be completely 2.0, but the idea should inform every decision made at the library.[4]

Dave King also views Library 2.0 through a technology lens:

Of course Library 2.0 is all about technology. But not technology for technology's sake. Not technology like silly, archaic, doesn't-really-make-sense-to-anyone-outside-the-library-world automation systems. The technology I'm talking about goes back to the concept of meeting your customers where they already are. Our patrons are using web 2.0 services. They are using cell phones. They are gaming, IM'ing, chatting. They are consuming digital content. And we as libraries need to be there, if we want to meet and greet our patrons.[5]

The true promise of 2.0 tools lies in content creation and the combination and reuse of applications in new and efficient ways. Other 2.0 applications, especially those related to social networking and virtual worlds, may have been overlooked because they are dominated by teenagers and young adults, and are viewed as standing apart from the realm of library operations. Web 2.0 technologies are characterized by peer production, mashups, social networking, syndication, and tagging. These resources function separately and collectively to form an interactive and sometimes immersive landscape as varied and diverse as their creators and inhabitants. Other authors in this volume delve into the particulars of the various technologies associated with this trend. This article will examine the potential impact of Library 2.0 on teaching and learning, in general, and medical libraries, in particular, and offer suggestions for incorporating 2.0 approaches sooner rather than later.

PEER PRODUCTION

Peer production refers to posting, subscribing, and tagging content in blogs, wikis, bookmarking sites, and other venues engaged in social networking. Composed of more than 50 million blogs and doubling in size every six months, the blogosphere features more than 2,000 scientific blogs that provide glimpses into scientific work and collaboration.[6] Peer production is not without its detractors. Some librarians without editing or uploading rights to their own library's Web content may question opening up read/write rights to patrons. Although some university libraries have been quick to establish a blog or wiki presence, in some cases, these resources appear as stodgy and uni-directional as static site content, with few comments from users. Some of these resources continue to tell (library hours) rather than involve (reviews, tags, subject guides). The more successful library blogs and wikis are lighthearted and promote a sense of community among a clearly defined or segmented population. Notable library wikis include the University of Connecticut's library staff wiki <http://wiki.lib.uconn.edu/wiki/Main_Page> and Library Success Wiki <http://www.libsuccess.org/index.php? title=Main_Page>, which focuses on best practices within the profession. A notable example outside the library realm includes RateMy Professors.com, which features candid assessment of college instructors. Rateyourstudents.blogspot.com was developed in reaction to RateMy Professors.com. Wikis and blogs of interest to scientific personnel include Clinical Cases and Images <http://casesblog.blogspot.com/>, Medicine Portal <http://en.wikipedia.org/wiki/Portal:Medicine>, and Flu Wiki <http://www.fluwikie.com/>. Boulos et al. have reported the usefulness of peer production in clinical settings.[7] A special issue of *Choice* focused on blogs in academia.[8]

MASHUPS

Originally spawned by the music industry, mashups combine existing applications to create unique, one-stop hybrid resources. Fichter provides a decent overview of the subject for librarians.[9] Many of the popular examples include map images from Google Maps <http://maps.google.com/>:

- **WeatherBonk** <http://www.weatherbonk.com/> combines weather forecasts; live weather conditions; seasonal highs and lows; temperature, radar, traffic, and satellite maps; and webcams for geographical locations across the nation.
- **Chicago Crimes** <http://chicagocrime.org/> combines online crime reports with street maps, satellite maps, and news reports.
- **Amazon's A9** <http://www.a9.com/> is a subsidiary of Amazon that searches a number of content segments (live.com, Amazon books,

Wikipedia, Web Booster, etc.) and cascades the results into side-by-side frames.

Other compelling tools have focused on adding value to PubMed by imparting meaning and context, including the following:

- **Collaborative Bio Curation** (CBioC) <http://cbioc.eas.asu.edu/> is a collaborative curation project developed by Arizona State University that uses a browser extension to extract salient information from PubMed abstracts and relate them to existing information in the cBioc database.
- **GoPubMed** <http://www.gopubmed.org/> uses a molecular biology structured vocabulary (Gene Ontology) to categorize PubMed abstracts. Features include semantic searching of genetic concepts, hot research topics, and editing an individualized ontology.[10]

A simple mashup is already in place at many medical libraries that use multi-protocol resources such as Trillian <http://www.download.com/3000-2150-10047473.html> or Pidgin Im <http://pidgin.im/pidgin/home> [Pidgin has subsumed Gaim] for instant messaging, regardless of the type of instant messaging system used by patrons.

SOCIAL NETWORKING

Social networking is a broad term that encompasses a variety of online activities including file sharing (text, images, music, audio, and video clips); online communities such as blogs, wikis, blikis (blog + wiki); communities of practice with common or segmented areas of interest (dating, high school reunions, dog owners, cat owners, professional networking, etc.); and virtual worlds that involve fantasy and role playing.[11] The interactivity sought and experienced by social networkers may be the closest to Berners-Lee's original notion of the Web as "the decentralized, organic growth of ideas, technology, and society."[12] The most popular social networking sites include MySpace, Facebook, Friendster, Bebo, Orkut, and Xanga. According to Nielsen/NetRatings, the top three social networking sites as of April 2006 were MySpace, Blogger, and Classmates Online.[13] The importance of one-stop resources and community as parts of the social environment cannot be underestimated.[14-19] Google's College Life <http://services.google.com/university/> is an example of an aggregated interface that combines Gmail, blogging, photo sharing,

Google Scholar, instant messaging, and SMS (short message service). Librarian Beth Evans reports that her daughter checks e-mail through MySpace and avoids her Hotmail because the daughter's friends do not send messages to her e-mail account.[20]

As defined by Gartner, social network analysis (SNA) can be used to better understand client groups.[21] How do people relate to each other and how does information flow between them? Librarians participating in social networks can analyze the characteristics and needs of their fellow networkers in efforts to improve library products and services, and create useful mashups.

Social networking tools have pervaded educational arenas.[22-25] The University of Pennsylvania's College Houses and Academic Services developed Pennster to create a sense of community among incoming first-year students.[26] This same idea can be applied to cohorts of new faculty, library staff, or students on clerkship rotations. Dickinson College in Carlisle, Pennsylvania hosts wikis and blogs for personal and/or instructional purposes. Dickinson's Mixxer <http://www.language-exhanges.org> connects native speakers with persons wishing to practice foreign language skills. A notable Dickinson wiki <http://itech.dickinson.edu/wiki/index.php/Toulouse_Study_Abroad_Program/> features student internship reports, information about excursions, and neighborhood research for students studying abroad. Community of Science (COS) <http://www.cos.com/> is a tool of enormous value to the scientific community at large. Established in 1989 at Johns Hopkins University, COS features 500,000 researcher profiles, searchable research interests, and sources of research funding.

SYNDICATION

Syndication refers to the pushing of content (text, images, audio, video) for immediate viewing/listening, downloading to another device, or delivery through an aggregator. This approach has replaced the notion of sticky site content by recognizing that it is more convenient to use a newsreader or feed aggregator to collect content from a variety of sources than to retrieve each individually. The most popular syndicated content includes updated blog/wiki/bliki entries, podcasts, vodcasts, and news feeds. Feed aggregators can be used to deliver automatic, updated content such as the latest table of contents from *Journal of Academic Librarianship*, search results from PubMed, or funding opportunities from the National Institutes of Health. Librarians can use an RSS feed aggregator to deliver tables of contents from the top ten publications cited by the organization's physicians, nurses, allied health professionals, researchers, and administrators, for example. Notable podcasting examples include the *New England Journal of Medicine* <http://podcast.nejm.org/> and the Cleveland Clinic <http://www.clevelandclinic.org/healthedge>. Brittain et al. describe their experience planning and creating podcasts of dental school lectures.[27]

TAGGING

Tagging refers to the addition of meaningful keywords to Web content (text, images, audio, video) for purposes of sharing, organization, and retrieval. Folksonomy is a term of recent vintage that describes this non-hierarchical and collaborative approach to tagging and sharing information.[28] The librarian who would rather search Google anew rather than sift through a long list of poorly organized browser bookmarks may not fully appreciate the value of shared bookmarks, even if supplemented by tags.[29] Notable examples include:

* **Dr. Steven L. MacCall's bookmarks on del.icio.us** <http://del.icio. us/ maccall>. Dr. MacCall teaches health sciences librarianship at the University of Alabama. His "favorites" list is tagged with terms from AAHSL (Association of Academic Health Sciences Librar- ies) to course names/topics (LS534_RSS or LS534_Social_Net- working) to Yahoo. Interested parties can subscribe to an RSS feed of updated content from his page.
* **Connotea** <http://www.connotea.org/> is an example of social bookmarking applied to scientific content.

Many resources that feature user-generated tags also depict the most common terms in a tag cloud formation (see Figure 1). The words in large font sizes are more common than other terms in the cloud.

VIRTUAL WORLDS

Digital games require skill with "pattern recognition, sense-making in confusing environments, and multi-tasking . . . [in the game world] . . . you immerse yourself in an immensely complex, information-rich, dynamic environment where you must sense, infer, decide, and act quickly."[30] Ac- cording to MMOGCHART.com, which tracks subscription growth of

FIGURE 1. Example of a Tag Cloud

social networking tag clouds RSS mashups

blogs file sharing **Medical Library 2.0**

learning wikis **born digital** immersion

folksonomy gaming peer production

Atom **read/write** virtual worlds **syndication**

interactivity Semantic Web

massively multiplayer online games (MMOGs), World of Warcraft (WoW) is the top game. More than 7 million persons have purchased WoW, an online, role-playing fantasy game that features races, classes, and professions of characters that form guilds to complete quests.[31, 32] WoW has been nicknamed "Warcrack" because of the addictive nature of the immersive experience.

Second Life <http://secondlife.com/> is another virtual environment that has received a great deal of press.[33, 34] As of November 26, 2006, this virtual place had a total of 1,636,578 residents, 631,795 of which were added in the previous 60 days, and 14,375 were currently logged in on a Sunday afternoon! Guus van den Brekel, a medical librarian in the Netherlands, is one of the librarians developing Medical Library 2.0 within Second Life.[35] The American Cancer Society recently partnered with Second Life to sponsor a series of fundraising events, but experienced some logistical problems handling the number of simultaneous donor participants.[36]

To experience a virtual world without paying software/subscription fees or downloading plugins, readers can look at Hive7 <http://wvw.hive7.com/>, which uses Ajax (Asynchronous JavaScript, XML, and cascading style sheets)[37] rather than Shockwave to create the interactive situations.

Scott Rice and Amy Harris at the University of North Carolina Greensboro Libraries developed an interactive, multiplayer game <http://library.uncg.edu/de/infolitgame.asp#> related to information literacy. It is not as immersive as some of the fantasy role playing games, but since it allows players to choose character images (or avatars) to play and compete, the game will hold appeal for typical undergraduate students. Because game-playing is popular among high school and college students, role playing and competition can be incorporated into library instruction.

WEB 3.0

Web 3.0 is a relatively new term that has been used to describe the Croquet Consortium <http://www.opencroquet.org/> and the Semantic Web. Croquet is an example of an interface that facilitates collaborative work processes by multiple users. Inexplicably, some recent reports[38] have "renamed" Semantic Web as Web 3.0 as if Web 2.0 was up and running, or passé, and in need of a patch or upgrade. In a nutshell, Semantic Web imparts meaning to existing Web content in order to improve automated searching and data mining functions.[39] For example, depending on context, the search term Magellan can mean many different things to different client groups. It can refer to Magellan the explorer, investment fund, global positioning system, spacecraft, and so forth. The University of Washington's KnowItAll <http://www.cs.washington.edu/research/knowitall/> project is an example of using data mining to find and collect reviews, an idea that has far-reaching implications for reviewing software, online resources, and much more.

DISCUSSION

Some readers may find that tools related to peer production, social networking, virtual worlds, and tagging cannot be applied or transferred readily to medical library settings. Because these tools have the power to transform teaching and learning, understanding how they function is essential to librarians providing existing services, and planning services and facilities for the future. In 2000, Lynch recommended that librarians define or redefine their own missions in light of the technological forces that were revolutionizing "teaching, learning, and research," requiring "a far different conception of the library . . . to respond to more nomadic and virtual clientele."[40]

In his description of new learning environments, Brown[30] states that "[t]oday's students want to create and learn at the same time. They want to put content to use immediately." For example, rather than submit course assignments by e-mail to the instructor, students can contribute work to a project wiki that can be restricted to students enrolled in the course. In this way, students can learn from each other and create meaningful and enduring content.

Since secondary schools and colleges have already capitalized on Web 2.0 technologies and adapted teaching and learning techniques to appeal to digital natives, these adaptations will eventually trickle down to the training of scientists, physicians, and allied health professionals, and ultimately affect medical library operations and facilities. Several authors, inside and outside the library world, have written compellingly on the perils and promise of next-generation library services.[41-44]

When Ludwig and Starr published their Delphi study in 2005, they reported that their study participants were cognizant of changes in "the way scientists communicate the results of their research," that would affect the design of library buildings.[45] Librarians and architects interested in library facility design also think about the library's relationship to its parent institution:

> As we go forward, we must recognize the meaningful contribution that the library can provide *if* planned correctly. The goal of effective planning is to make the experience and services of the library transparent to the user. Rather than hide resources, the library should bring them to the user, creating a one-stop shopping experience. Whether users access e-mail, digitized resources, or special print collections, or are reformatting and publishing a paper, the library should be the place to enable them to advance their learning experiences.[46]

The Institute of Medicine's *Academic Health Centers: Leading Change in the 21st Century* document forecasts a change in educational emphasis "toward . . . the needs of patients and populations and a focus on improving health."[47] To this end, in September 2006, the *New England Journal of Medicine* launched a new medical education series that will "engage the general readership . . . in a dialogue on the state of the art of medical education today."[48] American medical education reform has been a continual effort.[49] What, how, and when should physicians in training learn? The medical school at the University of Connecticut reduced classroom instruction time to implement "student continuity practice in which first- and second-year students are introduced to patients and follow them through their visits to doctors' offices."[50] This curricular change could easily benefit from the use of Web 2.0 technologies to track progress, share information, and connect with professors and patients, through a variety of mobile devices.

Scott Bennett points to a "move in higher education away from a teaching culture and toward a culture of learning," and mentions this shift's implications on the future of libraries and their operations.[51] Bennett goes on to suggest a more profound shift away from service toward learning. How do students learn? Which programs, services, facilities, and amenities foster a learning community within a library? Frischer proposes placing new activities such as virtual reality and immersive theaters in research libraries such as UCLA's Cultural Virtual Reality Laboratory (CVRLab) <http://www.cvrlab.org/>.[52] Other notable examples include the Texas Advanced Computing Center's Visualization Laboratory at the University of Texas at Austin <http://www.tacc.utexas.edu/resources/vislab/> and SPAWAR's Knowledge Wall <http://www.pacific-science.com/kmds/STRATMUS.htm>. The National Library of Medicine's long-range plan stresses the value of holographic immersion facilities to view and discuss diagnostic images of individual patients.[53] NLM also suggests making these resources accessible to K-12 students.

SUGGESTIONS

The amorphous and unclearly defined Library 2.0 has caused confusion within the profession and may threaten the comfort levels of librarians and library staff satisfied with the amount of existing workplace technology. Much has been written about how next-generation librarians have been excluded or discouraged, intentionally or unintentionally, from planning and decision-making.[54-56] Interestingly, some aspects of 2.0 technologies may make older generations of librarians feel marginalized, especially related to online virtual worlds and the stream of consciousness seen on many blogs. Serials librarian Eleanor I. Cook, for example, expresses admiration for the thinking and writing abilities of bloggers but suspects that many do not prepare or research topics to the extent that she does for the column she writes for *Against the Grain.*[57] In an effort to address learning issues related to newer technologies of the Library 2.0 ilk, the Public Library of Charlotte & Mecklenburg County <http://plcmcl2-about.blogspot.com/> developed a learning competition for library staff of all generations that involves expeirmenting with 23 things related to blogging, photo sharing, RSS feeds and newsreaders, generating images, tagging, wikis, open source productivity tools, sharing audio and video files, and much more. PLCMC library staff who successfully completed the 23 items by a specified date won a USB/MP3 player and qualified to win other prizes.

Many librarians pioneered the introduction of Internet applications and developed Gopher and Web sites in their organizations. Libraries function as the third place (not home, not office) for generations of no-madic clients. Readers can think about whether next year's cohort of li-brary users now lives in an online environment[58] and what he or she expects from the medical library.

If the online gaming world is too far afield from the mission and values of the institution, readers can try some ideas and approaches related to social networking, peer production, or syndication (see Table 1), or tag-ging (see Table 2). Mashups (see Table 2) may be worth exploring with information technology partners or consortial groups.

CONCLUSION

In 1994, Bill Gates is reported to have said that he saw "little com-mercial potential for the Internet for at least ten years." Sometimes it is difficult to spot trends from within the work trenches or to see applica-tions that can revolutionize aspects of everyday work. Library 2.0 is a significant sea of change that can be harnessed to expand into new ven-tures and adventures, to maintain medical librarians' stronghold as tech-nology leaders, and to fulfill the Web's original promise.

Technology continues to challenge and confound. Through it all, it is possible to find different and more efficient ways to perform routine tasks, and once in a great while, discover an entirely new way to be pro-ductive or creative. More than 30 years ago, Alvin Toffler observed that:

> Technology feeds on itself. Technology makes more technology possible, as we can see if we look for a moment at the process of innovation. Technological innovation consists of three stages, linked together in a self-reinforcing cycle. First, there is the creative,

TABLE 1. Library 2.0 Ideas–Social Networking, Peer Production, and Syndication

Social Networking
• **establish a profile on MySpace or Facebook to connect with potential library clientele** <http://myspace.com/utlibraries> • **incorporate gaming or virtual world concepts into library instruction** <http://library.uncg.edu/de/infolitgame.asp#> • **support gaming activities within the library** <http://www.library.uiuc.edu/gaming/>

Peer Production
• **replace staff intranet with a staff blog, wiki, or bliki** <http://wiki.lib.uconn.edu/wiki/Main_Page> • **develop blikis for journal clubs, clerkship rotations, service learning projects, etc.** <http://www.ganfyd.org/> <http://www.fluwikie.com/> • **use wiki/blog/bliki technology to develop subject guides or portals** <http://www.library.ohiou.edu/subjects/bizwiki/index.php/Main_Page> <http://www.libraryforlife.org/subjectguids/index.php/Main_Page> • **encourage users to rate library resources and services** <http://www.ratingzone.com/>

Syndication
• **develop podcasts of interest to clientele groups (lecture series, news updates, etc.)** <http://epnweb.org/> • **use RSS or Atom to syndicate site content to others** • **use feed aggregators or newsreaders to organize subscribed content** <http://www.bloglines.com/> <http://feeds.reddit.com/> • **use Flickr or Photobucket to organize library staff pictures, clip art, or pathology slides** <http://www.flickr.com/> <photobucket.com/>

feasible idea. Second, the practical application. Third, its diffusion throughout society. The process is completed, the loop closed, when the diffusion of technology embodying the new idea, in turn, helps generate new creative ideas. Today there is evidence that the time between each of these steps has been shortened.[59]

The concept of Library 2.0 is being diffused through conversation, discussion, and experimentation, much of it online. In summer 2006, Talis hosted a library mashup contest <http://www.talis.com> that resulted in incredibly creative and worthwhile entries. Medical librarians have long been valued for their knowledge and resourcefulness (see Figure 2).

The word "conversation" pervades discussions of the Web 2.0 and the Library 2.0 phenomena, as characterized by the thoughtful and insightful

TABLE 2. Library 2.0 Ideas–Mashups and Tagging

Mashups
• **use Trillian, Meebo, Pidgin or other multi-protocol system to aggregate instant messaging (Yahoo, MSN, AOL/AIM) for the purposes of chat reference** <http://www.lib.unc.edu/reference/imalibrariandavis.html>
• **use Google Maps to improve map and driving directions for library site, or combine staff library directory with building layouts or campus maps** <http://campusmaps.tamu.edu/> <http://www.cyris.us/proj/chimaps/libmap.php>
• **add book jackets and book reviews (published and user-generated) to OPAC and acquisitions lists** <http://www.hclib.org/catalog/>
• **create a mashup of peer institutions (latest news from each organization or pushpin map)** <http://news.google.com/> <http://www.google.com/apis/maps/>

Tagging
• **encourage users to add tags, reviews, and comments to catalog records; use this information to create hybrid products** <http://catalog.hclib.org/> <http://www.aadl.org/catalog>
• **create a tag cloud to represent RSS feeds** <http://tagcloud.com/>
• **create and tag a bookmark list to be shared with others** <http://www.squidoo.com/> <http://www.connotea.org/>

musings on blogs such as T. Scott <http://tscott.typepad.com/>, Library Garden <http://librarygarden.blogspot.com/>, and medinfo <http://medinfo. netbib.de/>. For hilarious sendups of library foibles, try Library Pariah <http://librarypariah.blogspot.com/>, an irreverent, multi-authored blog that blurs reality with parody, poking fun at user-developed subject guides, among other subjects.

One of Benjamin Franklin's many contributions includes the founding of Philadelphia's Library Company, the first subscription library in the United States. The setting of subscription fees was not intended to exclude but to share the costs of purchasing expensive books. Franklin's idea spread like wildfire, resulting in subscription libraries being established in many other cities, inspiring him to remark that "these Libraries have improved the general Conversation of Americans, made the common Tradesmen and Farmers as intelligent as most Gentlemen from other Countries." Readers can improve the institutional conversation by continuing to embrace change, reading the literature of other professional fields, understanding how and where learning takes place in the organization, and continuing to make the library a destination for real and virtual users alike.

FIGURE 2. "The Medical Librarian." *Bulletin of the Medical Library Association* 18, no. 1-2 (1929): 26-7.

BULLETIN OF THE MEDICAL LIBRARY ASSOCIATION

Edited by

JAMES F. BALLARD

Editorial Committee

Miss Blake Beem, Boston   Dr. H. E. MacDermot, Montreal
Dr. Charles F. Painter, Boston   Miss Mary Louise Marshall,
Dr. Henry R. Viets, Boston   New Orleans
Subscription $2 per year. Foreign countries $3. Single numbers $1.

Address all communications to the

Bulletin of the Medical Library Association, 8 Fenway, Boston, Mass.

Vol. XVIII   JANUARY-APRIL, 1929   No. 1-2

THE MEDICAL LIBRARIAN

The medical librarian was born with a silver answer under his tongue. Verily, thou shalt not phaze him. He hath a liberal education and acquireth knowledge daily. He knoweth the names of the readers and greeteth them. Sometimes he remembereth their middle initials. If a woman, she recalleth also their neckties and the color of their eyes.

The medical librarian must have the agility of a robin, the eye of a hawk and the voice of a dove. When he refuseth it seemeth like conferring a favor. He loveth his books. He handleth a rare old volume like a newborn babe. The waste of time is unknown to him. He knoweth that while he listeneth to a tedious recital he can figure where the money is coming from to mend that leak in the roof.

He is not disturbed when a wild-eyed youth cometh up to demand, "What use are eyebrows anyway?" He beginneth with the antennae of insects and worketh up. He may not be certain at the moment whether cachexia is a troublesome cough or a skin disease, but tomorrow he will know ALL about it, and henceforth thou shalt not stick him on cachexia. Frequently he hath disciples to whom he sayeth not merely, "Thou shalt do thus and so," but, "Thou shalt do thus and so, and I will explain to thee WHY." He is always approachable, and usually available, for though he roameth afar thou canst get him by phone. He taketh notes and is able to read them. He treasureth old clippings and pasteth them in books for reference. Even a toothache doth not affect his invariable courtesy. He putteth himself out for people and LIKETH it. He is just. His fellow-workers speak kindly of him at other times than just before Christmas or pay-day. His library looketh like a library and not like an art exhibit, curiosity shop, or a club room. People come there to read, and he seeth that not one goeth away empty handed. Search, and thou shalt find him, maybe even in thine own home town,

REFERENCES

1. Brown, John Seely. "Growing Up Digital: How the Web Changes Work, Education, and the Ways People Learn." *Change* 32, no. 2 (2000): 11-20.

2. O'Reilly, Tim. "What is Web 2.0: Design Patterns and Business Models for the Next Generation of Software." Available: <http://www.oreillynet.com/lpt/a/6228>. Accessed: November 22, 2006.

3. Houghton, Sarah. LibrarianInBlack.net. Available: <http://librarianinblack. typepad.com/librarianinblack/2005/12/library_20_disc.html>. Accessed: November 24, 2006.

4. Farkus, Meredith. "A TechSource Conversation with Meredith Farkas." Available: <http://www.techsource.ala.org/blog/2006/03/a-techsource-conversation-with-meredith-farkas.html>. Accessed: November 25, 2006.

5. King, Dave. Dave's Blog. Available: <http://daweed.blogspot.com/2005/12/why-library-20.html>. Accessed: November 25, 2006.

6. Gefter, Amanda. "This is Your Space." *New Scientist* 191, no. 2569 (September 16, 2006): 46-8.

7. Boulos, Maged N. Kamel; Maramba, Inocencio; and Wheeler, Steve. "Wikis, Blogs and Podcasts: A New Generation of Web-based Tools for Virtual Collaborative Clinical Practice and Education." *BMC Medical Education* 6, no. 41 (2006). Available: <http://www.biomedcentral.com/1472-6920/6/41>. Accessed: November 25, 2006.

8. Cohen, Laura B. "Blogs in Academia: A Resource Guide." *Choice: Current Reviews for Academic Libraries* special issue 43 (August 2006).

9. Fichter, Darlene. "Doing the Monster Mashup." *Online* 30, no. 4 (July/August 2006): 48-50.

10. Doms, Andreas, and Schroeder, Michael. "GoPubMed: Exploring PubMed With the Gene Ontology." *Nucleic Acids Research* 33 suppl. 2 (July 1, 2005). Available: <http://nar.oxfordjournals.org/cgi/reprint/33/suppl_2/W783>. Accessed: November 26, 2006.

11. Clemmitt, Marcia. "Cyber Socializing." *CQ Researcher* 16, no. 27 (July 28, 2006): 625-48.

12. Berners-Lee, Tim. *Weaving the Web*. San Francisco: Harper, 1999.

13. Nielsen/NetRatings. Available: <http://www.nielsen-netratings.com/>. Accessed: November 26, 2006.

14. Achterman, Doug. "Making Connections with Blogs and Wikis." *CSLA Journal* 30, no. 1 (2006): 29-31.

15. Abram, Stephen. "What Can MySpace Teach Us In School Libraries?" *Multimedia & Internet@Schools* 13, no. 4 (July/August 2006): 22-4.

16. Poftak, Amy. "Community 2.0: Introducing Social Networking for the Educational Set." *TechLearning* (August 15, 2006): 44. Available: <http://www.techlearning. com/story/showArticle.jhtml?articleID=191901615>. Accessed: November 24, 2006.

17. Walmsley, Andrew. "Social Interaction is Key to Web 2.0." *Marketing* (October 18, 2006): 13.

18. Warlick, David. "A Day in the Life of Web 2.0." *TechLearning* (October 15, 2006). Available: <http://www.techlearning.com/story/showArticle.jhtml?articleID=193200296>. Accessed: November 24, 2006.

19. Huwe, Terence K. "Social Networking Mixes the Hip with the Proven." *Computers in Libraries* 26, no. 10 (November/December 2006): 31-3.

20. Evans, Beth. "Your Space or MySpace." *NetConnect* (Fall 2006): 8-10, 12.

21. Gonsalves, Antone. "Gartner Names Hot Technologies With Greatest Potential Impact." *Information Week* (August 9, 2006). Available: <http://www.information week.com/internet/showArticle.jhtml?articleID=191900919>. Accessed: November 26, 2006.

22. Bryant, Todd. "Social Software in Academia." *EDUCAUSE Quarterly* 29, no. 2 (2006): 61-4.

23. Lackie, Robert J. "WEB 2.0 and Its Technologies for Collaborative Library Communication." *Multimedia & Internet@Schools* 13, no. 6 (November/December 2006): 9-12.

24. Salz, Peggy Anne. "Social Networking Tools: On The Road To Enlightenment." *EContent* 29, no. 8 (October 2006): 24-30.

25. Shanahan, Matt. "Bringing the Next-Generation Web to Science." *Scientific Computing* 23(October 2006): 22-3, 27.

26. Pennster. University of Pennsylvania, College Houses and Academic Services. Available: <http://www.rescomp.upenn.edu/pennster/>. Accessed: November 25, 2006.

27. Brittain, Sarah; Glowacki, Pietrek; Van Ittersum, Jared; and Johnson, Lynn. "Podcasting Lectures: Formative Evaluation Strategies Helped Identify a Solution to a Learning Dilemma." *EDUCAUSE Quarterly* 3 (2006): 24-31.

28. Dye, Jessica. "Folksonomy: A Game of High-tech (and High-stakes) Tag." *Econtent* 29, no. 3 (2006): 38-43.

29. Connor, Elizabeth. "Medical Librarian 2.0." *Medical Reference Services Quarterly* 26, no. 1 (Spring 2007): 1-15.

30. Brown, John Seely. "New Learning Environments for the 21st Century." *Change* 38, no. 5 (September/October 2006): 18-24.

31. Levy, Steven; Liu, Melinda; Croal, N'gal; and Tyre, Peg. "Living a Virtual Life." *Newsweek* 148, no. 12 (September 18, 2006): 48-50.

32. Metz, Cade. "Virtual World, Real Money: There.com Combines Social Networking With 3D-game Virtual Reality." *PC Magazine* 25, no. 18 (October 17, 2006): 60.

33. Jana, Reena, and McConnon, Ali. "Second Life Lessons." *Business Week* 4011 (November 27, 2006): 17, 24.

34. Steel, Emily. "Avatars at the Office: More Companies Move Into Virtual World 'Second Life'; Ugly Bosses Can Be Models." *Wall Street Journal* (November 13, 2006): B1.

35. Brekel, Guus van den. Available: <http://www.blogger.com/profile/5776149>. Accessed: November 27, 2006.

36. "Second Life Tip Sheet." *Business Week* no. 4011 (November 27, 2006). Available: <http://www.businessweek.com/magazine/content/06_48/b4011417.htm>. Accessed: November 27, 2006.

37. Clark, Jason A. "Building an Ajax Application from Scratch." *Computers in Libraries* 26, no. 10 (November/December 2006): 16-22.

38. Markoff, John. "Entrepreneurs See a Web Guided by Common Sense." *The New York Times,* November 12, 2006, Sunday edition, section 1: 1.

39. Weinberger, David. "The Case for the Two Semantic Webs." *KMWorld* (June 2006): 18-9.

40. Lynch, Clifford. "From Automation to Transformation." *EDUCAUSE Review* 35 (January/February 2000): 60-8. Available: <http://www.educause.edu/pub/er/erm00/pp060068.pdf>. Accessed: November 26, 2006.

41. Breeding, Marshall. "Technology for the Next Generation." *Computers in Libraries* 26, no. 10 (November/December 2006): 28-30.

42. Chad, Ken, and Miller, Paul. "Do Libraries Matter? The Rise of Library 2.0." Available: <http://www.talis.com/downloads/white_papers/DoLibrariesMatter.pdf>. Accessed: November 24, 2006.

43. Stephens, Michael. "Into a New World of Librarianship." *NextSpace: The OCLC Newsletter* 2(2006). Available: <http://www.oclc.org/nextspace/002/3.htm>. Accessed: November 23, 2006.

44. Notess, Greg R. "The Terrible Twos: Web 2.0, Library 2.0, and More." *Online* 30, no. 3 (2006): 40-2.

45. Ludwig, Logan, and Starr, Susan. "Library as Place: Results of a Delphi Study." *Journal of the Medical Library Association* 93, no. 3 (July 2005): 315-26.

46. Freeman, Geoffrey T. "The Library as Place: Changes in Learning Patterns, Collections, Technology, and Use." In *Library as Place: Rethinking Roles, Rethinking Space*. CLIR Report 129. Washington, DC: Council on Library and Information Resources, 2005. Available: <http://www.clir.org/pubs/reports/pub129/freeman.html>. Accessed: November 22, 2006.

47. Institute of Medicine. *Academic Health Centers: Leading Change in the 21st Century*. Available: <http://www.iom.edu/CMS/3809/4673/13728.aspx>. Accessed: November 24, 2006.

48. Cox, Malcolm, and Irby, David M. "A New Series on Medical Education." *New England Journal of Medicine* 355, no. 12 (September 28, 2006): 1375-6. Available: <http://content.nejm.org/cgi/content/full/355/13/1375>. Accessed: November 22, 2006.

49. Cooke, Molly; Irby, David M.; Sullivan, William; and Ludmerer, Kenneth M. "American Medical Education 100 Years After the Flexner Report." *New England Journal of Medicine* 355, no. 12 (September 28, 2006): 1339-44. Available: <http://content.nejm.org/cgi/content/full/355/13/1339>. Accessed: November 22, 2006.

50. Rajan, T. V. "Making Medical Education Relevant."*The Chronicle of Higher Education* 52, no. 19 (January 13, 2006).

51. Bennett, Scott. "Righting the Balance." In *Library as Place: Rethinking Roles, Rethinking Space*. CLIR Report 129. Washington, DC: Council on Library and Information Resources, 2005. Available: <http://www.clir.org/pubs/reports/pub129/ bennett.html>. Accessed: November 22, 2006.

52. Frischer, Bernard. "The Ultimate Internet Café: Reflections of a Practicing Digital Humanist About Designing a Future for the Research Library in the Digital Age." *Library as Place: Rethinking Roles, Rethinking Space*. CLIR Report 129. Washington, DC: Council on Library and Information Resources, 2005. Available: <http://www.clir.org/ pubs/reports/pub129/frischer.html>. Accessed: November 22, 2006.

53. National Library of Medicine Board of Regents. *Charting a Course for the 21st Century: NLM's Long Range Plan 2006-2016*. Bethesda, MD: U. S. Department of Health and Human Services, Public Health Service, National Institutes of Health, 2006. Available: <http://www.nlm.nih.gov/pubs/plan/lrpdocs.html>. Accessed: November 22, 2006.

54. Gordon, Rachel Singer. "Generational Journeys." *Library Journal* 130, no. 3 (February 15, 2005): 42.

55. DiGilio, John J., and Lynn-Nelson, Gayle. "The Millennial Invasion." *Information Outlook* 8, no. 11 (November 2004): 15-20.

56. Lancaster, Lynne C. "The Click and Clash of Generations." *Library Journal* 128, no. 17 (October 15, 2003): 36-9.

57. Cook, Eleanor. "Drinking from the Firehose–Blogs are Making Me Feel Old!" *Against the Grain* 18, no. 5 (2006): 64, 68.

58. Hinton, Andrew. "We Live Here: Games, Third Places and the Information Architecture of the Future." *Bulletin of the American Society for Information Science and Technology* 32, no. 6 (August/September 2006): 17-21.
59. Toffler, Alvin. *Future Shock.* New York: Random House, 1970.

doi:10.1300/J115v26S01_02

Virtual Reference Services for the Academic Health Sciences Librarian 2.0

Ana D. Cleveland
Jodi L. Philbrick

SUMMARY. Virtual reference services in academic health sciences libraries are fast becoming a popular way to deliver information services, as the results of the authors' study indicate. Over 90% of academic health sciences libraries offer virtual reference services with Web forms being the most common form of delivery. In the article, the authors provide an overview of virtual reference services, discuss key issues related to the provision of virtual reference services, review the literature on virtual reference services in academic health sciences libraries, and present a study on the trends in virtual reference services in academic health sciences libraries. doi:10.1300/J115v26S01_03 *[Article copies available for a fee from The Haworth Document Delivery Service: 1-800-HAWORTH. E-mail address: <docdelivery@haworthpress.com> Website: <http://www.HaworthPress. com> © 2007 by The Haworth Press, Inc. All rights reserved.]*

Ana D. Cleveland, PhD, AHIP (ana@lis.admin.unt.edu) is Professor and Director, Health Informatics and Houston Programs, School of Library and Information Sciences, University of North Texas, P.O. Box 311068, Denton, TX 76203-1068. Jodi L. Philbrick, MLS (wilcoxen@lis.admin.unt.edu) is Assistant Director, Houston Program, adjunct faculty, and doctoral candidate, School of Library and Information Sciences, University of North Texas, P.O. Box 311068, Denton, TX 76203-1068.

[Haworth co-indexing entry note]: "Virtual Reference Services for the Academic Health Sciences Librarian 2.0." Cleveland, Ana D., and Jodi L. Philbrick. Co-published simultaneously in *Medical Reference Services Quarterly* (The Haworth Information Press, an imprint of The Haworth Press, Inc.) Vol. 26, Supp. #1, 2007, pp. 25-49; and: *Medical Librarian 2.0: Use of Web 2.0 Technologies in Reference Services* (ed: M. Sandra Wood) The Haworth Information Press, an imprint of The Haworth Press, Inc., 2007, pp. 25-49. Single or multiple copies of this article are available for a fee from The Haworth Document Delivery Service [1-800-HAWORTH, 9:00 a.m. - 5:00 p.m. (EST). E-mail address: docdelivery@haworthpress.com].

Available online at http://mrsq.haworthpress.com
doi:10.1300/J115v26S01_03

KEYWORDS. Virtual reference services, e-mail, Web forms, chat, instant messaging, academic health sciences libraries

INTRODUCTION

Librarians are used to delivering reference services in-person and via postal mail, telephone, and fax. With the advent of the Internet, technologies such as electronic mail (e-mail) and chat were tapped to deliver information services to users. Using these technologies to communicate with users has changed the landscape of reference services. In this article, the authors will provide an overview of virtual reference services, discuss key issues related to the provision of virtual reference services, review the literature on virtual reference services in academic health sciences libraries, and present a study on the trends in virtual reference services in academic health sciences libraries.

OVERVIEW OF VIRTUAL REFERENCE SERVICES

Virtual reference services, digital reference services, electronic reference services, and online reference services are terms that have been used in the literature to describe the interaction between users and librarians using Internet technologies. As Lankes writes, all of the terms "share a central concept: the use of software and the Internet to facilitate human intermediation at a distance."[1] For the purposes of this paper, the term virtual reference services will be used.

It is interesting to note that although the terms mentioned above have been used in the literature, they are not necessarily the terms or phrases used to index the articles in popular library and information sciences and medical databases. For instance, a search in the thesaurus of *Library and Information Science Abstracts* yielded the phrase "Online reference work" to identify articles about virtual reference services, and the thesaurus of *Library Literature and Information Science Full-Text* uses the phrase "Reference services/Automation," which is used for "Automation of library processes/Reference services," "Online reference services," and "Virtual reference." Most interestingly, MeSH has no entry for virtual reference services or any variation of the phrase, and when conducting a search in PubMed on the topic, some articles were assigned the MeSH term of "Library Services/trends." Once again, this illustrates the lack of consistency in the terminology used for virtual reference services.

Just as there are many terms used for virtual reference services in the literature, there are many definitions of the concept. Markgren, Ascher, Crow, and Lougee-Heimer provide a general definition; "virtual reference, in the broadest sense, means nothing more than asking and answering a reference question via the Internet."[2] The Reference and User Services Association (RUSA), part of the American Library Association (ALA), defines virtual reference as a "reference service initiated electronically, often in real-time, where patrons employ computers or other Internet technology to communicate with reference staff without being physically present."[3] Another simpler definition offered by Lankes is "the use of human intermediation to answer questions in a digital environment,"[4] and this is similar to the definition given by Pomerantz, who states that it is "a service that provides users with answers to questions in a computer-mediated environment."[5] Jin, Huang, Lin, and Guo offer a more detailed definition of virtual reference and write that it "refers to delivering a library reference service by electronic means, from asynchronous via e-mail, Web form, to real-time via chat, Web push, co-browsing, Voice over IP, etc."[6]

As the last definition illustrates, there are two categories of virtual reference services: asynchronous and synchronous. Asynchronous reference services do not occur in real-time; examples include e-mail, Web forms, and short message service (SMS) text messaging via cell phones. Synchronous reference services occur in real-time; examples include chat, instant messaging (IM), videoconferencing, and Voice over Internet Protocol (VoIP).

Academic health sciences libraries primarily use e-mail, Web forms, chat, and IM to deliver reference services, and these forms of reference will be explored in more depth. As Gray writes, "Libraries began experimenting with e-mail reference services in the mid-1980s, mainly in health science and engineering libraries," and she attributes this to the fact that scientists and engineers were one of the first groups to use the Internet and e-mail.[7] Over twenty years later, e-mail continues to be the most common form of virtual reference services,[8] which is not surprising considering that "over 90% of [I]nternet users send and receive email."[9] Communication via e-mail can take several iterations if information requests or responses need clarification, which can make the process very time consuming. Also, users may not respond when asked for clarification, thereby ending the transaction. As Gross, McClure, and Lankes state, "the idea that users would provide formulated questions if they wrote them out has not generally turned out to be true," and "this realization eventually led to a second standard of service in which a

Web form interface is typically used to solicit specific information about questions from users and to limit digital reference requests to ready reference questions."[8]

Web forms, as mentioned previously, are an extension of e-mail, and they are online forms that users fill out and submit to the library. Web forms utilize fields that help to structure the user's information request. Janes and Silverstein's examination of Web forms revealed that nearly all Web forms have fields that ask for the user's name and e-mail address, and the next most popular fields were phone number, affiliation, and street/mailing address.[10] Asynchronous reference services, although popular, do not offer interactivity, so libraries started experimenting with synchronous reference services in the 1990s.

Literature about chat reference services began appearing in the late 1990s.[11] As Mon writes, "chats can be one-to-one, as with call center software used by many libraries, or one-to-many if chat room software connects many patrons with a librarian."[12] Depending on the features of the software being used, chats may also include co-browsing, Web pushing, and application sharing. These features can create a very rich environment for users and librarians, but at the same time, using these features requires users and librarians to have certain settings or plug-ins on their computer. Not having the appropriate settings or plug-ins may dissuade users from using the service. As Lupien writes, "it is difficult to determine how many users lack the technical expertise, patience, and/ or inclination to go through a configuration process or download a piece of software onto their computer," and "it is reasonable to assume that this has an important impact on usage."[13] Despite the technological drawbacks, librarians cannot overlook the fact that co-browsing is important to the instructional aspect of virtual reference, and as Graves and Desai report, it "can be an effective teaching technique" and was well-received by users despite the technical difficulties involved.[14] Also, Johnston, through her study on digital reference transcripts, found that "60 percent of queries contain some instructional element."[15] As discussed, chat reference service has advantages and disadvantages.

The three forms of virtual reference services mentioned earlier, e-mail, Web forms, and chat, can be offered through vendor-provided virtual reference software packages. Some of the more popular software packages are Tutor.com's Ask a Librarian, OCLC's QuestionPoint, Docutek VRL*plus*, and LivePerson Pro (see Table 1 for more information). Common features of these software packages include e-mail management, call alerts, pushing, co-browsing, escorting, queue management, knowledge bases, scripts, and post-chat surveys.[16,17] Although dated,

TABLE 1. Selected List of Virtual Reference Vendors and Their Products

Vendor	Product	Web Site
Tutor.com	Ask a Librarian	<http://www.tutor.com/products/aal.aspx>
OCLC	Question Point	<http://www.questionpoint.org/>
Docutek	VRL*plus*	<http://www.docutek.com/products/vrlplus/index.html>
LivePerson	LivePerson Pro	<http://www.liveperson.com/>

Hirko[18] and Olivares[17] provide useful information about the different virtual reference software packages available. According to Coffman, as of 2004, prices for high-end software packages can vary from $2,000 to $6,000 per "seat."[19] Due to the costs associated virtual reference software packages, libraries have formed consortia to help offset the costs,[20] and other libraries have experimented with open source chat reference software, such as RAKIM.[21] Also, some libraries have decided to forgo virtual reference software packages and have moved to other freely available alternatives to provide synchronous reference services, such as IM clients.

Libraries that decide to use IM to deliver reference services will be reaching a large audience of users. According to the Pew Internet and American Life Project, "42% of [I]nternet users–more than 53 million American adults–report using instant messaging," and "although most [I]nternet users favor email over IM as a form of communication, nearly a quarter of IM users say they instant message more than they email."[22] Instant messaging is a form of chat, and it "can provide both one-to-one or one-to-many synchronous conversations, usually text-based, although voice chat is also available."[11] Several free IM programs are available, including AOL Instant Messenger, MSN Messenger, Yahoo! Messenger, Google Talk, and ICQ. Trillian, an IM aggregator program, allows users to monitor several different IM accounts, and this is a useful tool for librarians who may offer IM reference service using different IM services. Another IM service is Meebo, which allows users to log into their IM accounts without having to download the IM client, and this is helpful for users who may be working away from their home computer. More information about IM services is available in Table 2. IM has its advantages as reported by Houghton and Schmidt in their comparison of IM and Web-based chat[23] and by Abram in his "Twenty Reasons to Love IM" article.[24] However, VanScoy's examination of IM found some disadvantages of this type of virtual reference service, including "privacy problems, reliability issues, the lack of automatically generated statistics, and the need for patrons to create accounts."[25]

TABLE 2. Selected List of Instant Messaging Services

Instant Messaging Service	Web Site
AOL Instant Messenger	<http://www.aim.com/>
MSN Messenger	<http://get.live.com/messenger/overview>
Yahoo! Messenger	<http://messenger.yahoo.com/>
Google Talk	<http://www.google.com/talk/>
ICQ	<http://www.icq.com/>
Trillian	<http://www.trillian.cc/>
Meebo	<http://www31.meebo.com/index-en.html>

Libraries must assess the needs of their users to decide what type(s) of virtual reference services to offer. Due to current trends in the use of information technologies, providing only one type of virtual reference service may not be enough. According to a recent AP-AOL poll, "almost three-fourths of adults who do use instant messages still communicate with e-mail more often," and "almost three-fourths of teens send instant messages more than e-mail."[26] In an effort to reach out to the millennials (ages 18-24) using IM, the University of Illinois at Urbana-Champaign Library pilot tested an IM reference service that would be offered simultaneously with their popular chat reference service, and Ward and Kern found that having both services enabled them to reach all types of users.[27] Libraries need to experiment with different types of virtual reference services in order to find the right combination of services that meet the demands of their users.

ISSUES IN DELIVERING VIRTUAL REFERENCE SERVICES

There are a multitude of issues to consider when delivering virtual reference services, and some of these issues, including communication, policies and guidelines, marketing, and evaluation, will be discussed.

Communication

Communication is an essential component of delivering reference services, no matter what modality is being used. Computer-mediated communication (CMC) has similarities to face-to-face communication, but there are inherent differences due to the technologies being used. CMC is conducted through written text, whereas face-to-face communication is conducted orally. As Nilsen writes, "virtual reference requires both the library staff member and the user to type out their responses," and "written messages provide no verbal cues and tone of voice is lost."[28] Nonverbal cues are also missing in written messages, and librarians cannot see the user's body posture, attentiveness, smiling, and frowning.[29] Emoticons can help portray these nonverbal cues, but they "provide a shallow substitute for these indicators."[29] Another element librarians need to keep in mind is that electronic communication gives users anonymity, and this "protects and emboldens troublemakers, putting librarians at a distinct disadvantage."[30]

Librarians need to develop the skills to communicate in a computer-mediated environment, and "even the most skilled reference librarians struggle to answer questions that normally do not pose any difficulty for them in face-to-face encounters because of the newly imposed limitations of communicating solely by the written word."[31] Ronan gives broad observations regarding communicating in chat and instant messaging, which can help provide a basis for librarians to understand the nature of the environment.[31] Also, another interesting element of Ronan's article is her application of the RUSA *Guidelines for Behavioral Performance of Reference and Information Services Professionals* to the chat environment,[31] and Bell and Levy also provide a critique of the *Guidelines* along with their ideas for augmentation for virtual reference services.[32]

Radford's application of communication theories to virtual reference services help librarians to understand how to improve virtual reference interviews.[33,34] The results of her study on interpersonal communication in chat reference showed that interpersonal skills important in face-to-face interviews are still used, but modified, in virtual reference services, and these skills are "rapport building, compensation for lack of nonverbal cues, strategies for relationship development, evidence of deference and respect, face-saving tactics, greeting and closing rituals."[34] Like Radford, Westbrook looks to theories in other disciplines, such as psychology, education, communication, and human-computer interaction, and she believes these should be incorporated into virtual reference training.[35]

Another element that librarians need to consider is the language that is used in the electronic environment. The language of electronic communication can be very informal and "requires the librarian to establish the professional tone even while using a conversational medium."[36] As Bobrowsky, Beck, and Grant write, it can be difficult to balance "the need for a certain degree for formality combined with the need to communicate quickly."[37] Also, librarians need to be aware of the common abbreviations that are used often in chat for faster communication, such as LOL (laughing out loud), BTW (by the way), and THX (thanks). To increase the speed of communication, it is easy for librarians to use canned or scripted messages during the virtual reference interview, but Straw advises that librarians need to use these messages cautiously and only when appropriate during the interview to maintain the human element of the interaction.[38] Overall, communication may have an impact in the success of the virtual reference services.

Policies and Guidelines

Policies and guidelines are an important element of offering virtual reference services. According to *Webster's New Collegiate Dictionary*, a policy is "a high-level overall plan embracing the general goals and acceptable procedures,"[39] and a guideline is "an indication or outline . . . of policy or conduct."[40] There are two major guidelines for virtual reference services: RUSA's *Guidelines for Implementing and Maintaining Virtual Reference Services*[3] and the International Federation of Library Associations and Institutions' (IFLA) *Digital Reference Guidelines*.[41] RUSA's *Guidelines for Implementing and Maintaining Virtual Reference Services* has five sections: (1) Definition of Virtual Reference, (2) Preparing for Virtual Reference Services, (3) Provision of Service, (4) Organization of Service, and (5) Privacy. IFLA's *Digital Reference Guidelines* has two major sections: Administration of Digital Reference Services and Practice of Digital Reference. Another set of guidelines is the *Facets of Quality for Digital Reference Services*, which "outlines the important characteristics and features . . . for building a digital reference service for all audiences," and it has two major sections: User Transaction and Service Development and Management.[42] All of these guidelines can help libraries write their own policies for virtual reference services.

As Kern and Gillie write, "policies are an important tool in communicating intentions and restrictions of our services," and they "are also valuable in managing services and maintaining consistency."[43] There are two types of policies: internal (for staff use) and publicly available.[44] Lipow lists ten elements that should be considered when writing policies for virtual reference: eligibility, confidentiality, use of licensed databases to answer questions, identifying yourself to the client, delivery of material to the client, average length of transaction, client satisfaction, inappropriate client behavior, questionable questions, limit of transactions per client, and follow-up.[44] It is always helpful to research other policies before developing a policy for virtual reference services. The Statewide Virtual Reference Project of the Washington State Library offers a listing of example policies and procedures, indicating which libraries address user service overview, privacy and rules of conduct, and staff guidelines.[45] Policies become more challenging for libraries working in a collaborative virtual reference service because virtual reference librarians need to be familiar with the general library policies of all the institutions involved. To assist member libraries' staff engaged in collaborative efforts, OCLC's QuestionPoint provides *Global Reference Network Guidelines*[46] and *24/7 Reference Collaborative Policies and Procedures*[47] for member libraries. In summary, "the most important challenge for virtual reference policy is to match the practice of service to the policy and match the policy to the mission."[43]

Marketing

Marketing is an important step in creating awareness of a virtual reference service. It is important to note that some libraries have been reluctant to market their virtual reference services due to a variety of reasons, such as being afraid that demand for the service will exceed their resources.

Meola and Stormont provide five different models (basic, homegrown, advanced, collaborative, and corporate) for marketing virtual reference services depending on the needs of the library.[48] Some of the issues that need to be considered when marketing a virtual reference service include the naming of the service (i.e., "Ask a Librarian" or "Contact Us"), the location of the link to the service, and using multiple formats to promote the service.

Naming of the virtual reference service is important because it needs to convey the purpose of the service to the users. Duncan and Fichter applied usability testing techniques in order to name their virtual reference service as well as determine the location of the links to their virtual reference service on the library's Web pages. Their results showed that "Ask a Librarian" was the best choice for the name and that the best location for a text link was the top of the middle column of links.[49] Wells' study shows the importance of placing the button or link for virtual reference services on heavily used library Web pages, so the library can deliver help when users need it.[50] Gray supports this notion by stating that the "placement on Web pages of links to electronic reference services, as well as the number of links to the service throughout the Web site, directly affects the amount of traffic a service can expect."[7]

Multiple formats should be used to market virtual reference services. One idea for marketing a service is using business cards, like the ones developed for the University of Wisconsin-Madison e-mail reference service.[51] The cards included the librarians' name and e-mail address along with a link to the library home page. Another more current way to market virtual reference services is to develop a MySpace account (or an account for a similar service, such as Facebook) for the library. Due to the "popularity and reach of this powerful social network, libraries have a chance . . . to bring their services to the public."[52]

Bailey-Hainer provides an excellent resource on marketing, which includes AskColorado's marketing communications strategy and plan that other libraries could adopt and a listing of marketing resources at the end of the article.[53] Also, the King County Library System and the University of Washington offer a comprehensive set of guidelines for marketing virtual reference services.[54] On a final note, creative approaches combined with aggressive marketing are key factors in creating successful virtual reference services.

Evaluation

Anytime a service is offered, it needs to be evaluated in order to see if it is meeting the needs of the users. Meola and Stormont describe a general process of evaluating virtual reference services that includes the following steps: (1) Revisit Your Vision, (2) Evaluate Software, (3) Assess Staffing, (4) Review Questions, (5) Analyze Answers, and (6) Produce a Report.[48] The Statewide Virtual Reference Project of the Washington State Library provides a comprehensive manual for evaluating virtual reference services that includes checklists for libraries to use.[55] Another extensive evaluation manual is *Statistics, Measures, and Quality Standards for Assessing Digital Reference Library Services* by McClure, Lankes, Gross, and Choltco-Delvin.[56] The *Facets of Quality*, mentioned previously as a set of guidelines, has also been used to measure the quality of virtual reference services.[42]

One method that many libraries use to evaluate their virtual reference services is to analyze the transcripts of the transactions. The transcripts and logs of virtual reference services provide rich data sets, which could be used to assess the effectiveness and efficiency of the service as well as provide a deeper understanding of the information behavior of users. However, librarians do have their reservations about transcript analysis because it means that others can review their work at the reference desk. Using transcripts, librarians can analyze how well a question was answered, which was the focus of a study by Arnold and Kaske to evaluate chat reference service.[57] Transcripts, because of the information they contain, raise privacy and confidentiality issues that libraries have to take into consideration.

Evaluation, especially from the user's perspective, has been one area of virtual reference that needs more exploration. Most of the evaluation of user satisfaction has been done using pop-up or linked surveys at the end of virtual reference transactions.[58] To help address this issue, Radford and Connaway were recently awarded a grant from the Institute of Museum and Library Services to study users' and librarians' satisfaction with virtual reference services.[59] Finally, more research in the area of evaluation in virtual reference services needs to be undertaken to gain a better understanding of the services virtual reference librarians are providing.

LITERATURE REVIEW:
VIRTUAL REFERENCE SERVICES
IN ACADEMIC HEALTH SCIENCES LIBRARIES

Academic health sciences librarians have been at the forefront of virtual reference services from the very beginning. According to Sloan,[60] one of the first articles on virtual reference services was "Reference Services by Electronic Mail" by Ellen H. Howard and Terry Ann Jankowski of the University of Washington Health Sciences Library; it was published 20 years ago in the January 1986 issue of the *Bulletin of the Medical Library Association*.[61] Following this publication, the October 1986 issue of the same journal also featured an article on e-mail reference service by Frieda O. Weise and Marilyn Borgendale of the University of Maryland at Baltimore (UMAB) Health Sciences Library.[62] Both of these articles described the implementation of e-mail reference services in academic health sciences libraries. More articles regarding this subject were published in the 1990s, including Fishman's discussion of planning e-mail reference services at UMAB[63] and Schilling-Eccles and Harzbecker's study on the use of e-mail reference services at Alumni Medical Library at Boston University Medical Center.[64]

In the past 20 years, other academic health sciences libraries have experimented with offering other types of virtual reference services. In 1997, the University of California-Irvine offered reference services via desktop videoconferencing to medical students working in a computer lab.[65] Beginning in the 2000s, chat was the next type of virtual reference service to be explored in the literature. Connor provides an overview of chat reference services, including chat, instant messaging, features of chat and call center technologies, issues and challenges, and examples.[66] The summer 2003 issue of the *Medical Reference Services Quarterly* was solely devoted to the topic of chat reference services. Dee opened the issue with an article that discusses management issues related to chat reference including chat reference software.[67] In addition, the issue featured articles on implementations of chat reference services at academic health sciences libraries at the University of California-Irvine,[68] Duke University,[69] and the University of North Carolina-Chapel Hill.[70] Academic health sciences libraries have also participated in collaborative virtual reference services, such as the project between the Denison Memorial Library at the University of Colorado Health Sciences Center and J. Otto Lottes Health Sciences Library at the University of Missouri-Columbia.[71] McClellan discusses the University of Medicine and Dentistry of New Jersey's Health Sciences Library at Stratford participation in the Q and A NJ, a statewide 24/7 interactive reference service.[72] Not all implementations of chat reference services have been successful. Bobal, Schmidt, and Cox discuss the McGoogan Library of Medicine at the University of Nebraska Medical Center's experience with chat reference services and how they decided to discontinue the service due to difficulties with the software and low usage statistics.[73] Dee and Newhouse's article on digital chat reference in health sciences libraries helps to make decisions about implementing virtual reference services, and it provides information about planning for new services, assessing user needs, selecting software, collaboration, and marketing.[74]

Another dimension on the literature of virtual reference services in academic health sciences libraries is the examination of questions that are received at the virtual reference desk. Powell and Bradigan studied the e-mail reference questions they received at the Ohio State University John A. Prior Health Sciences Library from 1995 to 2000. They put the questions into nine categories: access to online services, citation verification, consumer health, database searching advice, directory information, holdings information, library services, professional information, and statistical information.[75] In a similar study, Markgren, Ascher, Crow, and Lougee-Heimer looked at the types of e-mail questions received at two different academic health sciences libraries (Gustave L. and Janet W. Levy Library at the Mount Sinai School of Medicine and the Medical Sciences Library at the New York Medical College) using QuestionPoint. They found the questions fell into six categories: technical, access to electronic resources, research, research (related to home institution), ready reference, and request for new acquisition.[2] Not surprisingly, the authors of the study found that one difference in the questions received via e-mail was the lack of directional questions that are normally associated with the physical reference desk. DeGroote compared the types of questions asked at the physical reference desk versus the virtual reference desk, including both e-mail and chat, at the University of Illinois at Chicago Library of the Health Sciences.[76] In-person reference questions focused on journal holdings, book holdings, and technical/access issues; chat reference questions focused on how to find articles on a particular topic; and e-mail reference questions focused on journal holdings, media items, and finding articles on a particular topic.

Trends in virtual reference services in academic health sciences libraries has primarily been examined by Dee in two studies, one in 2002 and one in 2004.[77, 78] The latest study reported an increase in the number of academic health sciences libraries offering chat reference services. The majority of the libraries offer e-mail services only, and some do not offer any form of virtual reference services.

As the trends indicate, academic health sciences libraries are offering virtual reference services, and there is support in the literature that academic health sciences libraries should continue, if not increase, these types of services. For instance, Tao, Demiris, Graves, and Sievert identified the "provision of 'virtual reference services'" as one of the "critical areas that can improve libraries' services and enhance their transition from a 'warehouse' model to a dynamic service provider."[79] The explosion of electronic resources, including textbooks, databases, e-journals, and Web sites, in academic health sciences libraries has given users greater access to materials away from the library;[2] thus, there has become a need to reach users when they need help, creating a "point-of-need" service. The new generation of library users is increasingly more savvy using technology in their daily lives, and libraries should be ready to incorporate this technology into the delivery of their services. As a recent editorial in the *BMJ* expressed, "younger doctors are digital natives."[80] Also, according to the Pew Internet and American Life Project, 31% of teens use the Internet for health information, representing about six million people, and these individuals will grow up to be the future users of academic health sciences libraries.[81] Academic health sciences librarians cannot overlook how virtual reference services are capable of "supporting service learning activities at clinical sites, and staying in touch with visiting and rotating personnel."[65] As Gail Kouame stated, "Digital reference has become accepted as a standard form of interacting with patrons,"[82] and this reflects the trend in virtual reference services in academic health sciences libraries.

TRENDS IN VIRTUAL REFERENCE SERVICES IN ACADEMIC HEALTH SCIENCES LIBRARIES

To supplement the discussion of virtual reference services, the authors conducted a study of the current trends in virtual reference services in academic health sciences libraries in fall 2006. The authors examined the Web sites of the 137 academic health sciences libraries represented in the *Membership Directory of the Association of Academic Health Sciences Libraries* (AAHSL)[83] to answer the questions outlined below.

Questions Explored

- How many academic health sciences libraries offer virtual reference services?
- What types of virtual reference services do academic health sciences libraries offer?
- How do academic health sciences libraries label their virtual reference services?
- When do academic health sciences libraries offer their synchronous (chat or IM) virtual reference services?
- How many academic health sciences libraries place limits on who can use their virtual reference services?
- How many academic health sciences libraries have privacy policies for their virtual reference services?

Results

Academic Health Sciences Libraries Offering Virtual Reference Services

After analyzing the 137 Web sites of the academic health sciences libraries, the authors found that 127 (93%) academic health sciences libraries offer virtual reference services, and seven (5%) academic health sciences libraries do not offer virtual reference services. Three (2%) libraries did not have enough information available on their Web sites to indicate whether or not they offered virtual reference services.

Types of Virtual Reference Services Offered by Academic Health Sciences Libraries

Academic health sciences libraries offer four different types of virtual reference services: e-mail, Web forms, chat, and instant messaging. Of the 127 academic health sciences libraries that offer virtual reference services, 92 (72%) offer Web form-based reference services, 49 (39%) offer e-mail reference services, 35 (28%) offer chat reference services, and 30 (24%) offer IM reference services (see Figure 1). Also, 126 (99%) libraries offer asynchronous (e-mail or Web form) reference services, and 54 (43%) libraries offer synchronous (chat or IM) reference services.

In terms of what combinations of services the libraries are offering, 42 (33%) of the libraries *only* offer Web form-based reference service, and 22 (17%) *only* offer e-mail reference service. One library *only* offers chat reference service, and no libraries offer IM reference service by itself. More information about the combinations of virtual reference services offered by the academic health sciences libraries can be found in Figure 2.

Labeling of Virtual Reference Services by Academic Health Sciences Libraries

The majority of libraries (78 out of 127, or 61%) use the phrase "Ask a Librarian" (or derivatives, such as "Ask a Reference Librarian" or

FIGURE 1. Types of Virtual Reference Services in Academic Health Sciences Libraries

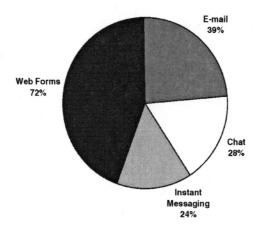

FIGURE 2. Combination of Virtual Reference Services in Academic Health Sciences Libraries

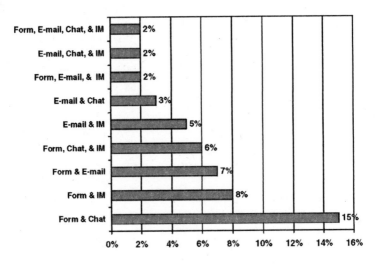

"Ask a HSL Librarian") as a label for their virtual reference services. Other examples of labels used are "Ask Us" or "Ask a Reference Question." In some cases, "Ask a Librarian" links to the whole suite of reference services the library offers, including face-to-face and telephone reference services, and in other cases, "Ask a Librarian" links directly to a particular type of virtual reference service that the library offers, such as a Web form.

When Synchronous Reference Services Are Offered

Fifty-four out of 127 (43%) of the academic health sciences libraries offer synchronous reference services. Nineteen out of 54 (35%) of academic health sciences libraries offer synchronous reference services Monday through Friday. Eleven (20%) libraries offer synchronous reference services every day of the week, and 10 (19%) libraries do not state when they offer synchronous reference services. Figure 3 shows a breakdown of the days of the week when synchronous reference services are offered. During weekdays, the libraries open their services anywhere between 7:30 a.m. and 12:00 p.m. and close their services anywhere from 3:00 p.m. to 12:00 a.m., but the more common hours of business are 9:00 a.m. to 5:00 p.m. On weekends, the services start later

FIGURE 3. Days of the Week When Academic Health Sciences Libraries Offer Synchronous Reference Services

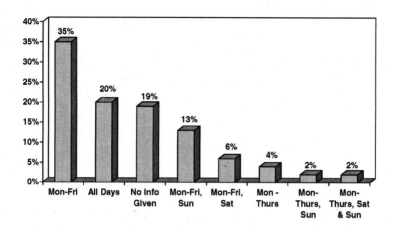

and end earlier. The number of open hours for virtual reference services ranges from two hours to 16 hours.

Limitations on Who Can Use Virtual Reference Services

Fifty out of 127 (39%) libraries place limitations on who can use their virtual reference services. Most libraries restrict their virtual reference services by including a statement that only affiliated users of their library may use the services. Ten out of the 50 (20%) libraries with limitations have password-protected services. One library used IP addresses to restrict access to their virtual reference services.

Privacy Policies for Virtual Reference Services

Thirty-six out of the 127 (28%) academic health sciences libraries offering virtual reference services have stated privacy policies and 18 out of the 36 (50%) libraries have policies that are directly related to their virtual reference services. The privacy policies of the remainder of the libraries are divided between library privacy policies (nine out of 36, or 25%) and university privacy policies (seven out of 36, or 22%). One library links to the *QuestionPoint Patron Terms of Service*, which includes a section on privacy.[84] Two libraries did not have policies, but they did provide statements about how they use transaction logs.

Discussion of the Study

The results of the authors' study show a rise in the number of libraries offering asynchronous and synchronous reference services compared to Dee's 2004 study.[78] Dee reports that 36 academic health sciences libraries offered chat reference services in 2004, and the results of the authors' study show that there are 54 libraries offering chat or IM reference services as of Fall 2006. Also, Dee reports that around 90% of libraries had e-mail reference services, and the authors' study indicates that 99% of libraries offer asynchronous reference services (e-mail or Web form). However, it is hard to make a direct comparison with Dee's study since the sample of the study is not clearly identified.

Labeling virtual reference services is always a daunting task, since it is important to create a name that properly indicates the purpose of the service to users. The results of the authors' study support Duncan and Fichter's finding that "Ask a Librarian" is a popular name for virtual reference services.[49] It is interesting to note that libraries are inconsistent in the terminology they use to identify their virtual reference services. For instance, they may label their IM reference service as "Chat" and label Web form-based reference service as "E-mail." As Heise and Kimmel note, this adds confusion to the users because the underlying software product is not identified when the service is named.[85]

The 2004 study by Dee reports that most libraries provided chat services Monday through Friday,[78] and this is consistent with the findings presented in the authors' study. Dee's study indicates that 27% of the libraries offered chat services during the weekend, and the authors' study shows an increase in this area as 23 out of 54 libraries (43%) offered synchronous reference services during the weekend. The hours of when synchronous reference services are offered are consistent with Dee's findings.

Kern and Gillie's study on virtual reference policies indicates that user restrictions were the most common policy element, and in several cases, libraries enforced the restrictions by requiring a special password or number to access the service.[43] Just over one-third (39%) of the academic health sciences libraries in this study place limitations on who can use their virtual reference services; half of these libraries do so by using password protections. Kibbee provides a good discussion of the issues academic librarians face in offering virtual reference services for unaffiliated users and gives practical advice on how to serve those users.[86]

RUSA's *Guidelines for Implementing and Maintaining Virtual Reference Services* suggest that "libraries need to develop . . . privacy policies for their virtual reference transactions."[3] The authors' study shows that relatively few libraries have privacy policies for their virtual reference services available on their Web sites. Through virtual reference transactions, librarians collect a lot of self-identifying information from virtual users that they do not collect from walk-in users,[87] and librarians need to think about the implications of storing and saving this kind of information about their users. Neuhaus reinforces the importance of privacy policies, and he outlines the information that should be included in a good privacy policy.[88]

In summary, the authors' study shows that academic health sciences libraries are increasing their use of virtual reference services. Most libraries are offering asynchronous reference services, but more libraries have added synchronous reference services. "Ask a Librarian" is the common name used to label virtual reference services in academic health sciences libraries. Libraries that offer synchronous reference services do so during weekdays during normal working hours. Some, but not a majority of academic health sciences libraries, place restrictions on who can use their virtual reference services. Privacy policies are an area that could be improved upon, as just over a quarter of libraries have policies available on their Web sites.

CONCLUSION

Currently, much is being said about the concept of Web 2.0, which is perceived as an evolution of Internet-based services focusing on the human aspects of Web interactivity. If this is a true characterization, then a corollary would be that Library 2.0, as a derivative, is focusing on the human aspects of library-based interactivity. The technologies used by many academic health sciences libraries to deliver virtual reference services are positioning health sciences librarians as a Librarian 2.0.

Discovering, learning, and applying new avenues of services to meet the information needs of their users have been a long tradition of academic health sciences librarians. Not surprisingly, academic health sciences librarians have been the pioneers of virtual reference services and continue to increase their offering of these services as the authors' study shows. In the future, the authors expect that academic health sciences librarians will continue to explore new ways to deliver virtual reference services, such as blogs, to meet the needs of their users.

There are major issues that academic health sciences libraries need to understand when offering virtual reference services. Consistency of the terminology, in terms of the concept, indexing, and labeling of services, is an area that needs improvement. Communication, policies and guidelines, marketing, and evaluation are management issues that are also vital to the success of virtual reference services.

From the exploration of the literature on virtual reference services in academic health sciences libraries, it is evident there is a need to continue to offer, if not increase, virtual reference services in academic health sciences libraries due to the present and future generations' patterns of technology use. It is encouraging to see that the majority of academic health sciences libraries are responding to the call for information at the point-of-need by offering virtual reference services.

REFERENCES

1. Lankes, R.D. "The Digital Reference Research Agenda." *Journal of the American Society for Information Science and Technology* 55, no. 4 (2004): 301-11.

2. Markgen, S.; Ascher, M.T.; Crow, S.J.; and Lougee-Heimer, H. "Asked and Answered–Online: How Two Medical Libraries are Using OCLC's QuestionPoint to Answer Reference Questions." *Medical Reference Services Quarterly* 23, no. 1 (Spring 2004): 13-28.

3. MARS Digital Reference Guidelines Ad Hoc Committee, Reference and User Services Association. "Guidelines for Implementing and Maintaining Virtual Reference Services." (2004). Available: <http://www.ala.org/ala/rusa/rusaprotools/referenceguide/virtrefguidelines.htm>. Accessed: October 28, 2006.

4. Lankes, R.D. "Digital Reference Research: Fusing Research and Practice." *Reference & User Services Quarterly* 44, no. 4 (Summer 2005): 320-6.

5. Pomerantz, J. "Integrating Digital Reference Service into the Digital Library Environment in the Digital Reference Research Agenda." In *Publications in Librarianship*, edited by R.D. Lankes, A. Goodrum, and S. Nicholson, 23-47. Chicago: Association of College & Research Libraries, 2003.

6. Jin, Y.; Huang, M.; Lin, H.; and Guo, J. "Towards Collaboration: The Development of Collaborative Virtual Reference Service in China." *The Journal of Academic Librarianship* 31, no. 3 (May 2005): 287-91.

7. Gray, S.M. "Virtual Reference Services: Directions and Agendas." *Reference & User Services Quarterly* 39, no. 4 (Summer 2000): 365-75.

8. Gross, M.; McClure, C.; and Lankes. R.D. "Assessing Quality in Digital Reference Services: An Overview of the Key Literature on Digital Reference." In *Implementing Digital Reference Services: Setting Standards and Making it Real*, edited by R.D. Lankes, C.R. McClure, M. Gross, & J. Pomerantz, 171-183. New York: Neal Schuman, 2003.

9. Pew Internet & American Life Project. "How Women and Men Use the Internet." (December 28, 2005). Available: <http://www.pewinternet.org/pdfs/PIP_Women_and_Men_online.pdf>. Accessed: October 10, 2006.

10. Janes, J., and Silverstein, J. "Question Negotiation and the Technological Environment." *D-Lib Magazine* 9, no. 2 (February 2003). Available: <http://www.dlib. org/dlib/february03/janes/02janes.html>. Accessed: October 25, 2006.

11. Pomerantz, J. "A Conceptual Framework and Open Research Questions for Chat-Based Reference Services." *Journal of the American Society for Information Science and Technology* 56, no. 12 (2005): 1288-302.

12. Mon, L. "Digital Reference and Ubiquitous Computing in the Classroom." *Knowledge Quest* 34, no. 3 (January/February 2006): 20-3.

13. Lupien, P. "Virtual Reference in the Age of Pop-up Blockers, Firewalls, and Service Pack 2." *Online* 30, no. 4 (Jul/Aug 2006) Available: <http://www.infotoday.com/ online/jul06/Lupien.shtml>. Accessed: September 1, 2006.

14. Graves, S.J., and Desai, C. "Instruction via Chat Reference: Does Co-Browse Help?" *Reference Services Review* 34, no. 3 (2006): 340-57.

15. Johnston, P.E. "Digital Reference as an Instructional Tool." *Searcher* 11, no. 3 (March 2003): 31-3.

16. Janes, J. "Live Reference: Too Much, Too Fast?" *Library Journal NetConnect* 127, no. 17 (Fall 2002): 12-4.

17. Olivares, O. "May: Virtual Reference Systems." *Computers in Libraries* 24, no. 5 (May 2004): 25-9.

18. Hirko, B. "Live, Digital Reference Marketplace." *Library Journal NetConnect* 127, no. 17 (Fall 2002): 16-7.

19. Coffman, S., and Arret, L. "To Chat or Not to Chat–Taking Another Look at Virtual Reference, Part 1." *Searcher* 12, no. 7 (July/August 2004). Available: <http:// www.infotoday.com/searcher/jul04/arret_coffman.shtml>. Accessed: September 9, 2006.

20. Peters, T.A. "E-Reference: How Consortia Add Value." *The Journal of Academic Librarianship* 28, no. 4 (July 2002): 248-50.

21. Carraway, S., and Payne, S. "Implementing RAKIM Open Source Chat Reference Software." *Computers in Libraries* 25, no. 5 (May 2005): 10-5.

22. Pew Internet & American Life Project. "How Americans Use Instant Messaging." (September 1, 2004). Available: <http://www.pewinternet.org/pdfs/PIP_Instantmessage_ Report.pdf>. Accessed: October 10, 2006.

23. Houghton, S., and Schmidt, A. "Web-Based Chat vs. Instant Messaging: Who Wins?" *Online* 29, no. 4 (July/August 2005): 26-30.

24. Abram, S. "Twenty Reasons to Love IM." *Information Outlook* 8, no.10 (October 2004): 40-2.

25. VanScoy, A. "Page Us: Combining the Best of In-Person and Virtual Reference Service to Meet In-Library Patron Needs." *Internet Reference Services Quarterly* 11, no. 2 (2006): 15-25.

26. Lester, W. "Poll: 'IM-ing' Divides Teens, Adults." Yahoo! News (December 8, 2006). Available: <http://news.yahoo.com/s/ap/20061208/ap_on_hi_te/instant_ messaging_ap_poll>. Accessed: December 8, 2006.

27. Ward, D., and Kern, M.K. "Combining IM and Vendor-based Chat: A Report from the Frontlines of an Integrated Service." *portal: Libraries and the Academy* 6, no. 4 (2006): 417-29.

28. Nilsen, K. "The Library Visit Study: User Experiences at the Virtual Reference Desk." *Information Research* 9, no. 2 (January 2004). Available: <http://informationr. net/ir/9-2/paper171.html>. Accessed: September 10, 2006.

29. Lee, I.J. "Do Virtual Reference Librarians Dream of Digital Reference Questions?: A Qualitative and Quantitative Analysis of E-Mail and Chat Reference."

Australian Academic & Research Libraries 35, no. 2 (June 2004). Available: <http://alia.org.au/publishing/aarl/35.2/full.text/lee.html>. Accessed: October 10, 2006.

30. Braxton, S. "Eeewww! My Patron Tried to Pick Me Up." *American Libraries* 36, no. 4 (April 2005): 30.

31. Ronan, J. "The Reference Interview Online." *Reference & User Services Quarterly* 43, no. 1 (Fall 2003): 43-7.

32. Bell, J.G., and Levy, A.P. "Making the Digital Connection More Personal." In *The Virtual Reference Experience: Integrating Theory into Practice*, edited by R.D. Lankes, J. Janes, L.C. Smith, and C.M. Finneran, 139-61. New York: Neal Schuman, 2004.

33. Radford, M.L. "Communication Theory Applied to the Reference Encounter: An Analysis of Critical Incidents." *Library Quarterly* 66, no. 2 (1996): 123-37.

34. Radford, M.L. "Encountering Virtual Users: A Qualitative Investigation of Interpersonal Communication in Chat Reference." *Journal of the American Society for Information Science and Technology* 57, no.8 (June 2006): 1046-59.

35. Westbrook, L. "Virtual Reference Training: The Second Generation." *College & Research Libraries* 67, no. 3 (May 2006): 249-59.

36. Chase, D. "Papa's Got a Brand New (Virtual) Bag: Real-Time Chat and Reference Discourse." *Electronic Journal of Academic and Special Librarianship* 6, no. 1-2 (Summer 2005). Available: <http://southernlibrarianship.icaap.org/content/v06n01/chase_d01.htm>. Accessed: November 11, 2006.

37. Bobrowsky, T.; Beck, L.; and Grant, M. "The Chat Reference Interview: Practicalities and Advice." *The Reference Librarian* no. 89/90 (2005): 179-91.

38. Straw, J.E. "Using Canned Messages in Virtual Reference Communication." *Internet Reference Services Quarterly* 11, no.1 (2006): 39-49.

39. *Webster's New Collegiate Dictionary*. s.v. "guideline."

40. *Webster's New Collegiate Dictionary*. s.v. "policy."

41. International Federation of Library Associations and Institutions. "IFLA Digital Reference Services Guidelines." Available: <http://www.ifla.org/VII/s36/pubs/drg03.htm>. Accessed: September 2, 2006.

41. Virtual Reference Desk (VRD). "Facets of Quality for Digital Reference Services." (2003). Available: <http://www.webjunction.org/do/DisplayContent?id=11811>. Accessed: September 3, 2006.

43. Kern, M.K., and Gillie, E. "Virtual Reference Policies: An Examination of Current Practice." In *The Virtual Reference Experience: Integrating Theory into Practice*, edited by R.D. Lankes, J.Janes, L.C. Smith, and C.M. Finneran, 165-84. New York: Neal Schuman, 2004.

44. Lipow, A.G. *The Virtual Reference Librarian's Handbook*. Berkeley: Library Solutions Press, 2003.

45. Statewide Virtual Reference Project, Washington State Library. "Policies and Procedures for Virtual Reference." Available: <http://vrstrain.spl.org/vradventure/textdocs/poliprogrid.htm>. Accessed: September 9, 2006.

46. OCLC QuestionPoint. "Global Reference Network Guidelines." (2005). Available: <http://www.questionpoint.org/policies/memberguidelines.html>. Accessed: September 9, 2006.

47. OCLC QuestionPoint. "24/7 Reference Collaborative Policies and Procedures." (2005). Available: <http://www.questionpoint.org/ordering/cooperative_guidelines_247rev3.htm>. Accessed: September 9, 2006.

48. Meola, M., and Stormont, S. "Starting and Operating Live Virtual Reference Services." New York: Neal-Schuman, 2002.

49. Duncan, V., and Fichter, D.M. "What Words and Where? Applying Usability Testing Techniques to Name a New Live Reference Service." *Journal of the Medical Library Association* 92, no. 2 (April 2004): 218-25.

50. Wells, C.A. "Location, Location, Location: The Importance of Placement of the Chat Request Button." *Reference & User Services Quarterly* 43, no. 2 (Winter 2003): 133-7.

51. Jesudason, M. "Outreach to Student-Athletes through E-mail Reference Service." *Reference Services Review* 26, no. 3 (2000): 262-7.

52. Evans, B. "Your Space or MySpace." *Library Journal NetConnect* 131(Fall 2006): 8-12.

53. Bailey-Hainer, B. "Marketing Virtual Reference Services: The AskColorado Experience." *Oregon Library Association Quarterly* 10, no.2/3 (Fall 2004): 12-8.

54. King County Library System & University of Washington. "Virtual Reference Services: Marketing Guidelines." (2002). Available: <http://www.secstate.wa.gov/library/libraries/projects/virtualRef/textdocs/MarketingGuidelines.pdf>. Accessed: September 6, 2006.

55. Statewide Virtual Reference Project, Washington State Library. "VET: The Virtual Evaluation Toolkit." (2004). Available: <http://vrstrain.spl.org/vradventure/textdocs/VETmanual.pdf>. Accessed: November 1, 2006.

56. McClure, C.R.; Lankes, R.D.; Gross, M.; and Choltco-Delvin, B. "Statistics, Measures, and Quality Standards for Assessing Digital Reference Library Services: Guidelines and Procedures." (2002). Available: <http://data.webjunction.org/wj/documents/11813.pdf>. Accessed: September 30, 2006.

57. Arnold, J., and Kaske, N. "Evaluating the Quality of a Chat Service." *portal: Libraries and the Academy* 5, no. 2 (2005): 177-93.

58. Nilsen, K. "Comparing Users' Perspectives of In-Person and Virtual Reference." *New Library World* 107, no. 1222/1223 (2006): 91-104.

59. OCLC. "Seeking Synchronicity: Evaluating Virtual Reference Services from User, Non-User, and Librarian Perspectives." Available: <http://www.oclc.org/research/projects/synchronicity/description.htm>. Accessed: November 2, 2006.

60. Sloan, B. "Twenty Years of Virtual Reference." *Internet Reference Services Quarterly* 11, no. 2 (2006): 91-5.

61. Howard, E.H, and Jankowski, T.A. "Reference Services via Electronic Mail." *Bulletin of the Medical Library Association* 74, no. 1 (January 1986): 41-4.

62. Weise, F.O., and Borgendale, M. "EARS: Electronic Access to Reference Service." *Bulletin of the Medical Library Association* 74, no. 4 (October 1986): 300-4.

63. Fishman, D.L. "Managing the Virtual Reference Desk: How to Plan an Effective E-Mail System." *Medical Reference Services Quarterly* 7, no. 1 (Spring 1998): 1-10.

64. Schilling-Eccles, K., and Harzbecker, Jr., J.J. "The Use of Electronic Mail at the Reference Desk: Impact of a Computer-Mediated Communication Technology on Librarian-Client Interactions." *Medical Reference Services Quarterly* 17, no. 4 (Winter 1998): 17-27.

65. Lessick, S.; Kjaer, K.; and Clancy, S. "Interactive Reference Service (IRS) at UC Irvine: Expanding Reference Service Beyond the Reference Desk." *ACRL Conference Proceedings*, 1997. Available: <http://www.ala.org/ala/acrlbucket/nashville1997pap/lessickkjaer.htm>. Accessed: September 12, 2006.

66. Connor, E. "Real-Time Reference: The Use of Chat Technology to Improve Point of Need Assistance." *Medical Reference Services Quarterly* 21, no. 4 (Winter 2002): 1-11.

67. Dee, C.R. "Chat Reference Services in Medical Libraries: Part 1–An Introduction." *Medical Reference Services Quarterly* 22, no. 2 (Summer 2003): 1-13.

68. Jerant, L.L., and Firestein, K. "Not Virtual, but a Real, Live, Online Interactive Reference Service." *Medical Reference Services Quarterly* 22, no. 2 (Summer 2003): 57-68.

69. MacDonald, M.H. "Planning, Implementing, and Using a Virtual Reference Service." *Medical Reference Services Quarterly* 22, no. 2 (Summer 2003): 71-5.

70. McGraw, K.A.; Heiland, J.; and Harris, J.C. "Promotion and Evaluation of a Virtual Live Reference Service." *Medical Reference Services Quarterly* 22, no. 2 (Summer 2003): 41-56.

71. Parker, S.K., and Johnson, E.D. "The Region 4 Collaborative Virtual Reference Project." *Medical Reference Services Quarterly* 22, no. 2 (Summer 2003): 29-39.

72. McClellan, C.S. "Live Reference in an Academic Health Sciences Library: The Q and A NJ Experience at the University of Medicine and Dentistry of New Jersey Health Sciences Library at Stratford." In *Virtual Reference Services: Issues and Trends*, edited by S. Kimmel and J. Heise, 117-26. New York: The Haworth Information Press, 2003.

73. Bobal, A.M.; Schmidt, C.M.; and Cox, R. "One Library's Experience with Live, Virtual Reference." *Journal of the Medical Library Association* 93, no. 1 (January 2005): 123-5.

74. Dee, C.R., and Newhouse, J.D. "Digital Chat Reference in Health Science Libraries: Challenges in Initiating a New Service." *Medical Reference Services Quarterly* 24, no. 3 (Fall 2005): 17-27.

75. Powell, C.A., and Bradigan, P.S. "E-Mail Reference Services: Characteristics and Effects on Overall Reference Services at an Academic Health Sciences Library." *Reference & User Services Quarterly* 41, no.2 (Winter 2001): 170-8.

76. DeGroote, S. "Questions Asked at the Virtual and Physical Health Sciences Reference Desk: How Do They Compare and What Do They Tell Us." *Medical Reference Services Quarterly* 24, no. 2 (Summer 2005): 11-23.

77. Dee, C.R. "Chat Reference Service in Medical Libraries: Part 2–Trends in Medical School Libraries." *Medical Reference Services Quarterly* 22, no. 2 (Summer 2003): 15-28.

78. Dee, C.R. "Digital Reference Service: Trends in Academic Health Science Libraries." *Medical Reference Services Quarterly* 24, no. 1 (Spring 2005): 19-27.

79. Tao, D.; Demiris, G.; Graves, R.S.; and Sievert, M. "Transition from in Library Use of Resources to Outside Library Use: The Impact of Internet on Information Seeking Behavior of Medical Students and Faculty." *AMIA 2003 Annual Symposium Proceedings* (2003): 1027.

80. Johnson, J.; Dutton, S.; Briffa, E.; and Black, D.C. "Broadband Learning for Doctors." *BMJ* 332 (June 17, 2006): 1403-4.

81. Pew Internet and American Life Project. "Teens and Technology." (July 25, 2005). Available: <http://www.pewinternet.org/pdfs/PIP_Teens_Tech_July2005web.pdf>. Accessed: October 10, 2006.

82. Clemmons, N.W., and Clemmons, S.L. "Five Years Later: Medical Reference in the 21st Century." *Medical Reference Services Quarterly* 24, no.1 (Spring 2005): 1-17.

83. Association of Academic Health Sciences Libraries. "Membership Directory." Available: <http://www.aahsl.org/new/about/directory.cfm?action=byinst>. Accessed: October 13, 2006.

84. OCLC. "QuestionPoint Patron Terms of Service." (2005). Available: <http://www.questionpoint.org/ordering/pdfs/userterms/88561_170728.htm>. Accessed: November 1, 2006.

85. Heise, J., and Kimmel, S. "Reading the River: The State of the Art of Real-Time Virtual Reference." In *Virtual Reference Services: Issues and Trends*, edited by S. Kimmel and J. Heise, 1-7. New York: The Haworth Information Press, 2003.

86. Kibbee, J. "Librarians without Borders? Virtual Reference Service to Unaffiliated Users." *The Journal of Academic Librarianship* 32, no. 5 (September 2006): 467-73.

87. Sen-Roy, M. "The Social Life of Digital Reference: What the Technology Affords." *The Reference Librarian* 85 (2004): 127-37.

88. Neuhaus, P. "Privacy and Confidentiality in Digital Reference." *Reference & User Services Quarterly* 43, no. 1 (Fall 2003): 26-36.

doi:10.1300/J115v26S01_03

Applications of RSS
in Health Sciences Libraries

Alexia D. Estabrook
David L. Rothman

SUMMARY. RSS is a syndication technology based on XML. RSS can be used for current awareness and as a SDI tool for clinicians and information professionals alike, delivering syndicated information as it becomes available from blogs, databases, and other online information sources. RSS can also be used to create dynamic content on health sciences library Web sites. With a great number of free tools available, RSS can be integrated into library services simply and seamlessly, enhancing library service offerings at extremely low cost to health sciences libraries. doi:10.1300/J115v26S01_04 *[Article copies available for a fee from The Haworth Document Delivery Service: 1-800-HAWORTH. E-mail address: <docdelivery@haworthpress.com> Website: <http://www.HaworthPress.com> © 2007 by The Haworth Press, Inc. All rights reserved.]*

Alexia D. Estabrook, MSLS, AHIP (alexia.estabrook@providence-stjohnhealth. org) is Information Services Librarian, Providence Hospital, St. John Health, Helen L. DeRoy Medical Library, 16001 West Nine Mile Road, Southfield, MI 48075. David L. Rothman (david.rothman@gmail.com) is Information Services Specialist, Community General Hospital of Greater Syracuse, 4900 Broad Road, Syracuse, NY 13215.

David Rothman is a co-creator of LibWorm and the owner of the site davidrothman. net, both of which are discussed in this paper.

[Haworth co-indexing entry note]: "Applications of RSS in Health Sciences Libraries." Estabrook, Alexia D., and David L. Rothman. Co-published simultaneously in *Medical Reference Services Quarterly* (The Haworth Information Press, an imprint of The Haworth Press, Inc.) Vol. 26, Supp. #1, 2007, pp. 51-68; and: *Medical Librarian 2.0: Use of Web 2.0 Technologies in Reference Services* (ed: M. Sandra Wood) The Haworth Information Press, an imprint of The Haworth Press, Inc., 2007, pp. 51-68. Single or multiple copies of this article are available for a fee from The Haworth Document Delivery Service [1-800-HAWORTH, 9:00 a.m. - 5:00 p.m. (EST). E-mail address: docdelivery@haworthpress.com].

KEYWORDS. RSS, Really Simple Syndication, Rich Site Summary, RDF Site Summary, current awareness, selective dissemination of information, SDI, XML, World Wide Web, Internet, professional development

INTRODUCTION

A librarian's role is multifaceted. Among the many functions of a librarian is that of current awareness and selective dissemination of information (or SDI). The Internet has expanded the number of resources available to librarians and their patrons exponentially, threatening to overwhelm the librarian or clinician who attempts to stay on top of current developments in his or her field. Fortunately, the Internet has also given librarians a tool that helps deliver this information in a format that allows the user to view the information when, where, and how he or she wishes. This tool is RSS.

PART I:
DEFINITIONS, OVERVIEW,
AND REVIEW OF THE LITERATURE

Definitions

What is RSS? There is no universally accepted standard meaning for the acronym. RSS can stand for "RDF (Resource Description Framework) Site Summary," "Rich Site Summary" or, most popularly, "Really Simple Syndication." Technically speaking, RSS is "an XML document format used to distribute headline and other web content."[1] RSS was first developed by Netscape® in 1999 and is known today as RSS 0.91. Although officially obsolete, this version is extremely simple and therefore popular, especially among novice RSS creators. Another advantage of this version is that it can be easily migrated to version 2.0. RSS version 0.91 has evolved into RSS 2.0 via versions 0.93, 0.93 and 0.94 (now obsolete), and is owned by Userland. Version 2.0 is recommended for sites that require metadata-rich syndication. Lastly, RSS version 1.0, owned by RSS-DEV Working Group, is RDF-based and recommended for sites that use RDF-based applications. Atom is a syndication format that tends to be lumped together with RSS, but while it is an XML-based syndication format, it was developed to fix perceived shortcomings of RSS. Although RSS and Atom differ significantly, the difference between them is invisible to the average consumer of feeds.

"RSS in its natural state is meant for computers to process, not for people to read."[2] RSS uses XML (eXtensible Markup Language), which was created to describe and structure data. RSS is a specific type of XML document that breaks down information into smaller parts. Those parts are then reformatted into either a feed aggregator to be read at a later time or fed through a script and placed on a Web page. The former describes individuals pulling information to themselves; the latter is used to push information to individuals. The creation and exporting or publishing of RSS content is called syndication.[3]

An RSS aggregator is "software that collects and stores RSS feeds for you to read immediately or at your convenience."[3] Sometimes referred to as a "news reader," "feed reader," or simply a "reader," an aggregator takes the RSS feed and reformats it into a human-readable format. This involves parsing, which is the processing of XML data. Depending on the feed and the aggregator, the information is either presented in an abbreviated format that requires the user to go to the site to read the rest of the article, or the article is shown in full by the aggregator.

There are three major types of aggregators: Web-based aggregators, Desktop-based aggregators, and Web browser-based features or plugins. Perhaps the most important consideration when determining which type to use is the level of portability the user requires.

Web-based aggregators like Bloglines <http://www.bloglines.com/> or Google Reader <http://www.google.com/reader/> offer the advantage of being extremely portable. Because the user's account and feed subscriptions are saved on a Web server, the aggregator can be accessed from any computer with an Internet connection and a Web browser. This allows the user, for instance, to check feeds from home in the morning, and then check them again that afternoon from work without losing or duplicating posts.

Desktop-based aggregators that are installed on the user's computer are not portable but can offer more features and customization options. Web browser-based aggregators, either native features of the browser or plug-ins, can be portable if launched from a USB thumb drive. Feeds may also be read on mobile devices using a mobile content service such as Avantgo <http://www.avantgo.com> or a mobile version of a Web-based aggregator.

If a user wishes to avoid using aggregators but still wants to take advantage of frequently updated feeds, the user can subscribe via one of many services that will convert RSS feed contents to e-mail, instant messages, or SMS, including Rmail <http://www.r-mail.org/>, RSSFWD <http://www.rssfwd.com/>, Squeet <http://squeet.com/home.aspx>, FeedBlitz <http://www.feedblitz.com/>, FeedBurner <http://www.feedburner.com/>, and ZapTXT <http://zaptxt.com/>. Why would a library want to turn feeds into e-mail subscriptions? At the Samaritan Health Services libraries of central Oregon, Hope Leman wanted to have one Web site where her library's patrons could subscribe to an e-mailed table of contents for each journal to which the library had immediate full-text access. Using FeedBurner, she created an e-mail subscription form for each and built MedGrab <http://www.medgrab.com/>, which serves exactly this purpose.

Why RSS?

As early as 10 years ago, e-mail notification was touted as the wave of the future in terms of current awareness and SDI. While e-mail notification has its strong points, keeping up via aggregators does have advantages. Reading feeds via an aggregator does not clog up e-mail boxes. Subscribing to RSS feeds does not subject the user to the risk of spam (although some feeds do contain advertising). Aggregators show the user new content from Web sites automatically, saving readers the time and effort of finding new content themselves. Feeds can be scanned when convenient and don't get lost in the shuffle among other e-mails (or visa versa). Items are retrieved en mass and can be scanned collectively, whereas updates via e-mails are retrieved individually and must be located among the myriad other e-mails in an inbox. In addition, subscribing to an RSS feed is anonymous, requiring the disclosure of no personal information, not even an e-mail address. Subscription is controlled by the subscriber, not the content provider, so unsubscribing is easy and immediate.

RSS also offers advantages for webmasters and content managers. Using RSS, XML, and other features on Web sites, current information can be brought in from other sources automatically and embedded in Web sites. This offers an easy way to keep content current on a library Web site with minimal effort. Content pages can be created by anyone in the library by using social bookmarking sites, such as del.icio.us <http://del.icio.us>, and their RSS features to embed a list of subject-specific URLs onto a Web page. This eliminates the need for funneling changes to a subject page through a webmaster, thus allowing changes and additions to go live on a site more quickly. RSS "is a means of organizing and simplifying current awareness efforts."[4]

Who Provides RSS Feeds?

Major news media outlets and bloggers were amongst the first to offer RSS feeds. CNN <http://www.cnn.com/services/rss/>, The Motley Fool® <http://www.fool.com/About/Headlines/Rss.htm?source=LN&display= sitemap>, and Wired <http://feeds.wired.com/wired/topheadlines> led the field in RSS offerings. Today, the major news syndicates, newspapers, television news stations, and news magazines offer feeds for current news stories, often broken down into categories for more focused use. Government agencies and institutes, such as the National Institutes of Health <http://www.nih.gov/news/feed.xml> and the United States Department of Health and Human Services <http://www.hhs.gov/rss/news/hhsnews.xml>, offer feeds for news, announcements, and podcasts. Also, be sure not to miss the NLM's feeds for Clinical Alerts and Advisories <http://www.nlm.nih.gov/databases/alerts/clinical_alerts.html>. For a complete listing of Federal RSS feeds, see FirstGov.gov's page on RSS feeds <http://www.firstgov.gov/Topics/Reference_Shelf/Libraries/Podcast_RSS.shtml>. Some aggregators, such as Bloglines, offer ways to read listserv e-mails via RSS feeds. Social software sites such as del.icio.us and flickr(TM) have feed capabilities, wiki changes can be tracked, reminders and calendars can be delivered via feeds, podcasts can be monitored, packages can be tracked, comics can be read, traffic can be monitored, and weather can be provided all in one place–the aggregator.

Libraries, database vendors, and OPAC vendors are joining the RSS bandwagon. Libraries are developing feeds for their news and announcements. The Ann Arbor District Library <http://www.aadl.org> offers feeds of new fiction, non-fiction, and "hot reads," for example. RefWorks allows users to save bibliographies in XML to be used as RSS feeds. OPAC companies have integrated RSS into their products. Database vendors (EBSCO and PubMed, for example) allow searches to be saved as RSS feeds to be placed in aggregators.

Review of the Literature

A review of the literature on RSS can be broken down into three basic categories: (1) general information and overviews, (2) articles that discuss different projects that can be done by libraries, and (3) articles that summarize projects that were done by specific libraries. Searches were run in EBSCO Health Business Fulltext Elite; MEDLINE®; CINAHL®; Library, Information Science & Technology Abstracts (LISTA), and Google™ <http://www.google.com> using the following terms: RSS, Real Simple Syndication, Rich Site Summary, and RDF Site Summary.

The most comprehensive article containing general information and overviews of RSS is found on the World Wide Web. The RSS Compendium <http://allrss.com> offers information on every aspect of RSS, from directories and editors to readers and validators.[5] Information Pizza <http://www.nhmccd.edu/Templates/Content.aspx?pid=59927> is a tutorial-based resource created by Luke Rosenberger, Technology Librarian for North Harris Montgomery Community College District. Initially used as a staff development tool, Mr. Rosenberger posted the tutorial on the Web for the benefit of all.[6] Because these resources are on the Web, they are dynamic and evolve as the information evolves. The RSS Compendium does offer RSS feeds that allow users to track changes and additions to the site.

Traditional print articles are less comprehensive yet still very helpful. David Mattison's article on RSS gives a succinct overview of RSS from beginning to end, and how it relates to blogging and news feeds.[3] Susanne Bjorner's article in the November/December 2003 issue of *The CyberSkeptic's Guide to Internet Research* is a brief and excellent overview of RSS as a current awareness tool.[7] Fran Wilkie summarized a series of workshops on RSS,[8] and Karen Bannan talks about some issues to consider when adding feeds as content on Web sites.[9] Bryan Bergeron penned an article on RSS geared to the physician.[10]

A great deal of the literature found outlines a basic overview of RSS and offers ideas of how libraries can use RSS feeds to enhance services. Darlene Fichter wrote two articles on using RSS to create dynamic content on the library Web site.[1,2] Steven Cohen and Carol Cooke offer articles on using RSS for current awareness.[4,11] Barbara Schloman and Jack Yensen write articles to nurses regarding RSS as a current awareness tool, but the ideas could easily be incorporated into the library setting.[12,13] Lastly, Paul Pival's article on RSS and syndicated content offers many options and links to tools to add feeds to library Web sites.[14]

Several articles outline specific projects completed by libraries using RSS technologies. Kevin Broun discusses how his library combines RSS and e-mail to help familiarize patrons with the concept.[15] In a separate article, Broun writes about LION (LIbrary Online) that combined a database with RSS technology to push content to their patrons.[16] Paoshan Yue and Araby Greene write about their library's creation of an index of their journals that offer RSS feeds.[17] Qin Zhu talks about HP Labs Research Library's management of technical reports using metadata and RSS feeds.[18] Finally, Gillian Crawford writes about the TOCRoSS (Table of Contents by Really Simple Syndication) project funded by JISC.[19]

PART II:
TECHNIQUES AND TOOLS FOR USERS
PULLING INFORMATION FROM RSS FEEDS

RSS feeds can serve many needs in a medical library, including current awareness and professional development for library staff and consumer health news updates for patients, their families, and the community served by the medical library. It is especially helpful in expanding current awareness and SDI services for clinicians. In addition, syndication can facilitate content management aspects of Web site development.

Librarianship Current Awareness and Professional Development

Current Awareness

Library staff can subscribe to table of contents feeds from many library and information science journals. While some journals offer feeds from their own Web sites, many do not. Where they do not, feeds can often be generated from database services. For example, EBSCO Megafile and PubMed both contain the bibliographic records for *Medical Reference Services Quarterly*, so a "Journal Alert" can be set up from EBSCO creating an RSS feed that will alert library staff when new articles are available from *Medical Reference Services Quarterly*, or a journal title search can be created in PubMed and the results can be saved as an RSS feed and added to an aggregator for seamless updating.

SDI

While tables of contents are an excellent method of serendipitous discovery (finding the information you didn't know you needed), it is also useful for medical library staff to create searches on specific topics in databases that index LIS journals and output the search results as a feed. For example, a search can be run in PubMed that searches MEDLINE for information on medical librarianship and delivers it to your aggregator. A search in PubMed with the search string, *"Libraries, Medical" [MAJR],* results in an instant SDI alert when the results are saved as a feed and is an easy way to stay up-to-date on newly-published articles on medical libraries. For instructions on how to output a PubMed search as an RSS feed, see <http://www.nlm.nih.gov/pubs/techbull/mj05/mj05_rss.html> and <http://davidrothman.net/2006/07/17/how-to-generate-a-custom-rss-feed-from-pubmed/>. PubMed also recently updated its instructions on how to output search results as an RSS feed <http://www.nlm.nih.gov/bsd/pubmed_tutorial/m3017d.html>.

One of the most dynamic and exciting ways for library staff to stay on top of issues impacting the profession may be to subscribe to the feeds of librarianship blogs. There are a great number of excellent blogs about librarianship (collectively, they are often referred to as the "biblio-blogosphere"), including a significant number that specialize in issues facing medical/health sciences libraries. A list of medical librarianship blogs can be found at <http://liswiki.org/wiki/Medlib_Blogs>, a page of the LISwiki <http://liswiki.org> which lists (at the time of this writing) 33 blogs about medical librarianship, including their feeds. Also available at this site is an OPML file containing the feeds for each blog on the list. This OPML file can be easily imported into most aggregators to allow the user to subscribe to all of these blog feeds quickly and easily. OPML will be discussed in some detail later in this article.

Another way to find and receive information on new developments in librarianship via feeds is to visit LibWorm <http://www.libworm.com>. LibWorm indexes about 1,400 feeds of information by, for, about, or of interest to librarians, and any search performed at LibWorm can be outputted as an RSS feed. Medical librarians should search for "medical" or "health sciences" at LibWorm and can then subscribe to the results to stay on top of conversations on medical librarianship in the biblio-blogosphere and beyond. LibWorm also has pre-set searches and feed categories of interest to medical librarians, including feed categories Medical Libraries <http://www.libworm.com/rss/index.php/Medical-Libraries/ 12/> and Medical Librarianship <http://www.libworm. com/rss/index.php/Medical-Librarianship/11>, as well as a "Medicine" Subject search which attempts to collect most discussion of health topics discussed online among library professionals and paraprofessionals <http://www.libworm.com/rss/search.php?qu=medicine+medical+biomedicine+biomedical+%22health+sciences%22+%22health+science%22&t=Medicine&r=Any&o=d&f=c>.

Clinical Applications

Current Awareness

"The unprecedented access to up-to-the minute information from seemingly infinite online sources has redefined medical research, practice and education."[10] Librarians can assist clinicians in navigating the mire of medical information by teaching them how syndication tools can help them acquire the information they most need when they need it and how they want to read it. Historically, medical journals were the main means to disseminate new clinical and scholarly information. This largely holds true today, but syndication can offer a more automatic and less intrusive method for physicians to receive notification of new journal issues. Many medical journals now offer RSS feeds for their tables of contents, and links for these can usually be found somewhere on the front page of a journal's Web site. The links can be identified by the orange icons reading "XML," "RSS," or a square orange icon (see Figure 1), or links saying "subscribe" or "syndication." One of the best ways to find feeds offered by medical journals is to visit one of a number of directories that exist for this purpose, three of which are RSS4medics <http://www. rss4medics.com/directory.htm>, Medical Feeds <http://www.medical feeds.com>, and the NHS Feed Directory <http://www.library.nhs.uk/rss/ directory/Default.aspx>. Librarians should also consider adding links to table of contents RSS feeds to "A to Z" journal lists or link resolvers. (see Figure 2).

Some journals, however, don't offer RSS feeds for the tables of contents. In these circumstances, an RSS feed can be created from PubMed by following these instructions:

1. Navigate to PubMed <http://www.pubmed.gov/>.
2. Click on the *Limits* tab.
3. Click the *Add Journal* button.
4. Type in the name of the journal.

FIGURE 1. Syndication Feed Icons

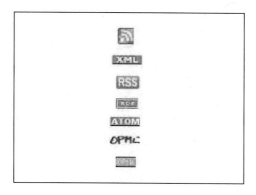

FIGURE 2. Example of RSS Feed Added to A to Z Journal Entry

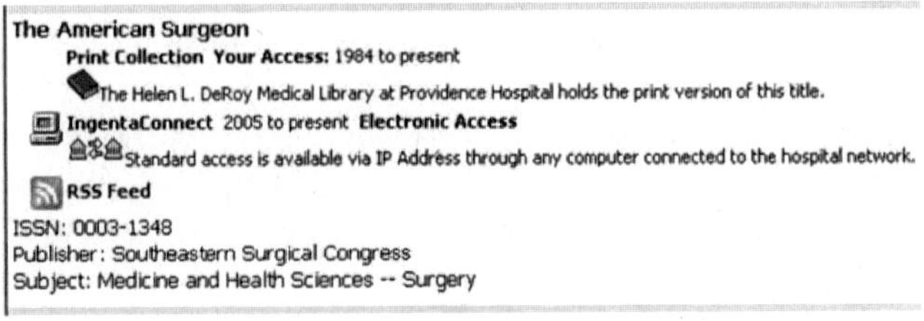

5. Scroll down to the bottom of the page and click the *Go* button.
6. Go to the *Send to* drop-down menu and select *RSS Feed*.
7. At *Limit Items if more than*, choose *50*.
8. Click *Create Feed* button.
9. Click on the orange XML button and copy and paste the URL from the address bar into your favorite aggregator.

Note: If you are using Firefox 2.0 or Internet Explorer 7, just clicking the XML button or link will allow you to quickly subscribe to the feed in the aggregator of your choice. Further details on using the feed-handling capabilities of Firefox 2.0 and Internet Explorer 7 are available at <http://davidrothman.net/2006/10/30/how-to-set-up-one-click-feed-subscription-in-firefox-20/> and <http://davidrothman.net/2006/10/30/how-to-set-up-one-click-feed-subscription-from-ie7-to-bloglines/> respectively. Further detail and illustrations on creating a table of contents feed from PubMed can be found at <http://davidrothman.net/2006/07/19/how-to-create-an-rss-feed-for-a-feedless-journal-with-pubmed/>.

SDI

Probably the most vital RSS-related service a medical library can provide to a clinician patron is to assist the patron in the creation of a PubMed query tailored to match specifically the current awareness needs of that patron (at the time this article was written, OVID did not offer the ability to save searches as RSS feeds, although they were working on it). Once the librarian is satisfied with the appropriateness of a query and the relevance of its results, the librarian only has to follow steps 6 through 9 from the instructions outlined earlier in the article to have the query run every day and output the results to an RSS feed.

Training Tools and Ideas

There are a great number of aggregators available for use, and no library can hope to be expert in the use of all of them. In order to ensure that the library can support the needs of patrons, it may be advisable for the individual library to designate one or two aggregators that it will support. Two good choices might be Bloglines and Google Reader, as both are Web-based aggregators that can be accessed from any Internet-connected computer. Both are powerful, flexible, and easy to use. Either one will allow the patron to mark an item to read later or to e-mail the item to a colleague or the library in order to request the article's full text. A list of potentially appropriate aggregators is given in Appendix A.

In addition, the library should also consider pre-configuring aggregators for patrons. The library could perform a quick interview with the patron to determine his or her needs, create the account with the designated aggregator, and set up subscriptions to the appropriate feeds on behalf of the patron. This, combined with the use of a Web-based aggregator, may allow library staff to directly assist with the patron's feed and aggregator questions or problems without the patron having to physically visit the library.

Another way to make receiving this information as convenient as possible for patrons is to encourage them to make use of notification tools. Bloglines has a free notifier <http://www.bloglines.com/about/notifier> that the patron can download that will inform him or her when new items are available through the feeds to which he or she is subscribed. If the patron uses Outlook 2007, he or she can have the convenience of reading his or her feeds in Outlook as well. If the patron is using an earlier version of Outlook, he or she may wish to consider downloading and installing one of these free plug-ins for Outlook that enable Outlook to handle feeds: RSS Popper <http://rsspopper.blogspot.com/2004/10/home.html>, BlogBot for Outlook <http://blogbot.com/out/>, Inclue! <http://www.inclue.com/home/>, and intraVnews <http://www.intravnews.com/>.

OPML

OPML stands for Outline Processor Markup Language and is an XML format for outlines. One of the uses that OPML has evolved into is for the exchange of lists of RSS feeds between aggregators. Lists of blogs with common themes can be saved as OPML files, as can feeds of journal tables of contents for medical specialties. This would allow the user to subscribe to many feeds at once. Most aggregators allow for easy subscribing to OPML files via an import feeds function. Creating the files is also easy. Bloglines and Google Reader both offer an export feature that allows the user to export the user's feeds as an OPML document. Opmlmanager <http://www.opmlmanager.com> is a Web-based OPML editor and hosting service. Once the OPML files are created, links can be placed on Web sites. Any additions or subtractions from the list would take place from the back end and no additional changes to the Web site are necessary.

PART III:
TECHNIQUES AND TOOLS
FOR PUSHING RSS FEEDS TO USERS

Displaying Feed Contents on a Web Page

Why would one want to display the contents of feeds on a library's Web site? Imagine being able to keep a continually updated page of news on any and every medical specialty. The library could have a "Gastroenterology News" page that would constantly show the most recent abstracts from the most important journals of the specialty. The library could even have its own news page on specific medical conditions, and could tweak the appearance of these automatically updating pages to match the appearance of the rest of the site. New acquisition lists are another way RSS feeds can be embedded into a Web page to include dynamic content. If a library's OPAC is not RSS capable, LibraryThing <http://www.librarything.com> can be used to create a feed. LibraryThing even offers a "widget" that helps users configure the script to add to their Web site.

Publishing a feed on a Web site requires an intermediate script that takes the raw RSS data and converts it to display on the site. There are several tools, both Web-based and server-based, that will accomplish this. When choosing a tool to publish feed contents to a Web site, the first consideration is whether to use a free, Web-based tool, or a free tool that the library must host for itself. The former tends to be easier to use, but may contain advertising. Another concern with the tools not hosted by the library is that Internet start-ups are born and die every day. A library shouldn't be so dependent on a Web-based tool that if it were to fold, the library's dependent services would end. On the other hand, solutions the library would host itself can be comfortably available as long as the library wants, but tend to be not quite as easy to use. The use of either requires little knowledge of HTML or scripting languages, but a hosted solution does require access to the institution's Web server. IT departments in hospitals tend to frown heavily upon downloading anything from the Web onto hospital servers and rarely give anyone outside the IT department access to configure anything on those servers; therefore, a Web-based tool may be the only option for the hospital librarian. Scripting tools are listed in Appendix B.

Filtering or Mashing Feeds

Some circumstances may call for the library to filter a feed, either including or excluding items based on pre-set criteria. For example, one might subscribe to a feed about gastroenterology, but only want to see items that mention Crohn's Disease. A feed filtering service like FeedShake <http://www.feedshake.com/> can take the publisher's feed, screen out the items that don't meet the criteria, and output a feed containing only those items that do meet the criteria.

Other circumstances may call for combining the contents of two or more feeds into a single feed. For example, a medical librarian might wish to simplify the subscription process for patrons by creating a single feed that contains all of the items from the tables of contents of multiple journals within a particular specialty so that any time a new clinician is being set up with an aggregator, the clinician or librarian can subscribe to just one feed that includes all of these. A good number of free tools exist to help do these things. For a list of Web-based feed filtering or mashing tools, see Appendix C.

Social Bookmarking and RSS

A medical library staffer will often run across items online that he or she wishes to share with clinicians, and it would be handy to be able to quickly and easily distribute these items to the interested individuals. Del.icio.us <http://del.icio.us> is one of several online social bookmarking applications that allows the user not only to bookmark Web pages in order to find them later, but to apply descriptive tags to those pages. One of the most useful applications of this is that del.icio.us can output as RSS any items given a particular tag by a particular user. If, for instance, one wanted to know when David Rothman bookmarked a site with the tag "google," one could subscribe to the following RSS feed: <http://del.icio.us/rss/david.rothman/google>. This same idea could be easily applied to an efficient means of distributing information to clinicians. The library could create a del.icio.us account and use only a previously agreed-upon list of tags, including those for medical specialties (e.g., cardiology, gastroenterology), for job titles (e.g., physician, RN, respiratory_therapist), or for hospital departments (e.g., senior_ management, radiology, physical_plant). A medical librarian could even use del.icio.us or FURL <http://www.furl.net/> to annotate Web resources using the controlled vocabulary of MeSH.

Tagging sites on social bookmarking sites is an easy way to include the entire library staff in Web content development regardless of their experience. As long as tagging is standardized and consistent, anytime a staff member finds a site that is appropriate to add to a subject page, the site can be tagged and will automatically show up on a page that has the appropriate RSS feed script. This eliminates the need for a content manager to make additions for everyone and significantly shortens the time from site discovery to placement on the Web site.

Creating Feeds for Web Pages That Have None

Sometimes there are pages that are regularly updated and do not offer RSS feeds. In these circumstances, several tools exist to allow the user to create an RSS feed from a Web page by demonstrating to the tool what items the user wants put into a feed. Of these, PonyFish <http://www.ponyfish.com/> is perhaps the easiest and most intuitive to use, while Feed43 <http://feed43.com/> may be among the most powerful. Other tools of the same type include WotzWot <http://www.wotzwot. com/>, FeedYes <http://www.feedyes.com/>, Feedfire <http://www. feedfire.com/>, Feedwhip <http://www.feedwhip.com/>, and Feedity <http://www.feedity.com/>.

The Future of RSS Feeds in Medical Libraries

Some vendors are now starting to sell RSS servers and services that allow a central administrator to control aggregator accounts, and this functionality would be enormously useful to libraries. The library staff could create subscriptions and make mass changes to subscriptions across the entire user base or a subsection thereof. New technologies and services powered by RSS are being created every day, and there is no predicting exactly what the future will bring, but the personalized nature of RSS feeds generated from custom search queries seems to be one of only a few available means of staying informed without being buried in the growing information avalanche.

CONCLUSION

RSS is a multifaceted tool that can be used in many aspects of knowledge management. The need for technical knowledge is minimized by the great and growing number of tools on the Web being developed for RSS. RSS can facilitate efficient professional development and current awareness in librarianship. Adding RSS content to a Web site, developing individual feeds for clinicians, and adding table of content feeds to A to Z lists are straightforward ways to enhance library services with minimal effort and maximum rewards. With RSS feeds being produced from everything from online calendars to blogs to wikis to social bookmarking tools, it's easy to start with a small project and add features and content as time and learning curves permit. As these syndication technologies evolve and gain support among publishers and medical information service providers, familiarity with their use will become increasingly important for medical library staffers.

REFERENCES

1. Fichter, D. "Using RSS to Create New Services." *Online* 28, no. 4 (2004): 52-5.

2. Fichter, D. "Always Fresh–Keeping Your Web Site Current with News Feeds." *Information Outlook* 10, no. 4 (2006): 27-9.

3. Mattison, D. "So You Want to Start a Syndicated Revolution: RSS News Blogging for Searchers." *Searcher: The Magazine for Database Professionals* 11, no. 2 (February 2003): 38-48.

4. Cooke, C.A. "Current Awareness in the New Millennium: RSS." *Medical Reference Services Quarterly* 25, no. 1 (Spring 2006): 59-69.

5. RSS Compendium. Available: <http://allrss.com>. Accessed: November 29, 2006.

6. Information Pizza. Available: <http://www.nhmccd.edu/Templates/Content.aspx?pid=59927>. Accessed: November 29, 2006.

7. Bjorner S. "RSS–Rich Site Summary." *Cyberskeptic's Guide to Internet Research* 8, no. 10 (November-December 2003): 1-2.

8. Wilkie, F. "Making Sense of RSS." *Health Information on the Internet* (August 2005): 5.

9. Bannan, KJ. "RSS: Lo-Fi Content Syndication." *ECONTENT* 25, no. 1 (January 2002): 31-3.

10. Bergeron, BP. "RSS Feeds: What are They and Why Should I Care?" *Journal of Medical Practice Management* 21, no. 6 (May-June 2006): 345-7.

11. Cohen, S.M. "Using RSS: An Explanation and Guide . . . Rich Site Summary." *Information Outlook* 6, no. 12 (December 2002): 6, 8, 10.

12. Schloman, B.F. "Information Resources. Staying Current: What RSS Can Do for You . . . 'really simple syndication' . . . 'rich site summary.'" *Online Journal of Issues in Nursing* 11, no. 1 (2006): 3.

13. Yensen, J. "Leveraging RSS Feeds to Support Xurrent Awareness." *CIN: Computers, Informatics, Nursing* 23, no. 3 (May-June 2005): 164-7.

14. Pival, P.R. "Moving Day: Making the Most of Your Message with RSS and Syndicated Content." *Feliciter* 52, no. 2 (2006): 62-5.
15. Broun, K. "Integrating Internet Content . . . RSS Feeds." *Library Journal; NetConnection* (Fall 2003): 20-3.
16. Broun, K. "New Dog, Old Trick: Alerts for RSS Feeds." *Library Journal; NetConnection* (Summer 2004): 18, 20.
17. Paoshan, Y.; Greene, A.; and Blackwell, L. "Do You See RSS in Your Future?" *Serials Librarian* 50, no. 3/4 (2006): 305-10.
18. Zhu Q. "THE NUTS AND BOLTS of Delivering New Technical Reports via Database-Generated RSS FEEDS." *Computers in Libraries* 26, no. 2 (2006): 24-8.
19. "Table of Contents by Really Simple Syndication." *Multimedia Information & Technology* 32, no. 3 (2006): 79-81.

FURTHER READING

Cohen, S.M. "Anyone Can Use an Aggregator." *Information Today* 23, no. 3 (2006): 23-5.
Connor, E. "Medical Librarian 2.0." *Medical Reference Services Quarterly* 26, no. 1 (Spring 2007):1-15.
Dempsey, K. "Librarians are Getting Pushy." *Computers in Libraries* 26, no. 2 (2006): 4.
Estabrook, A.D. "Technology. Leveraging Real Simple Syndication for Current Awareness." *Journal of Hospital Libraries* 5, no. 3 (2005): 83-92.
Fingerman, S. "Ready Reference–Blogs and RSS." *Cyberskeptic's Guide to Internet Research* 9(October 2004): 8.
Houghton, S. "Big Tech for Every Library." *Library Journal; NetConnection* 131 (Summer 2006): 12-5.
Jacobs, J.R. "RSS: It's Only XML But I Like It." *DttP* 32, no. 2 (2004): 10-1.
Mattison, D. "RSS News Blogging for Searchers." *Searcher* 11, no. 2 (February 2003): 38-48.
Miller, R. "RSS Right AND Wrongs." *EContent* 29, no. 7 (2006): 24-8.
Notess, G.R. "RSS, Aggregators, and Reading the Blog Fantastic." *Online* 26, no. 6 (November/December 2002): 52-4.
O'Neill, J. "Reference Point: RSS." *NFAIS Newsletter* 45, no. 1 (January-February 2003): 3.
"How to Explain RSS the Oprah Way." (2006). Available: <http://cravingideas.blogs.com/backinskinnyjeans/2006/09/how_to_explain_.html>. Accessed: December 5, 2006.
Tennant, R. "Digital Libraries. Feed Your Head: Keeping Up by Using RSS." *Library Journal* 128, no. 9 (May 15, 2003): 30.
Thomas, D. "RSS, Ruby, & the Web." *Dr Dobb's Journal* (2005): 26-30.
Weaver, B. "Coming, Ready or Not: RSS." *Online Currents* 18, no. 10 (December 2003): 3, 4, 6-8.
Winship, I. "Weblogs and RSS in Information Work." *Library and Information Update* 3, no. 5 (May 2004): 30-1.
Wu, W, and Li, J. "RSS Made Easy–A Basic Guide for Librarians." *Medical Reference Services Quarterly* 26, no. 1 (Spring 2007): 37-50.

doi:10.1300/J115v26S01_04

APPENDIX A

Aggregators

RSS Compendium-RSS Readers
<http://allrss.com/rssreaders.html>

A Directory of RSS Aggregators
<http://www.aggcompare.com/>

Comprehensive List of Aggregator Options
<http://www.newsonfeeds.com/faq/aggregators>

APPENDIX B

RSS Scripting Tools

Web-Based RSS-to-Web-Page tools

BlinkBits
<http://www.blinkbits.com/feed/build.php>

Feedo Style
<http://www.feedostyle.com/>

Feedroll
<http://www.feedroll.com/rssviewer/>

FeedSweep
<http://www.howdev.com/products//feedsweep/create_adv.asp>

RapidFeeds
<http://www.rapidfeeds.com>

RSS to JavaScript
<http://www.rss-to-javascript.com/>

RSSxpress-Lite
<http://rssxpress.ukoln.ac.uk/lite/include/?t=1>

Some Hosted RSS-to-Web-Page Tools

Feed2JS
<http://feed2js.org/>

JSMFeed.pl
<http://www.creativyst.com/Prod/18/>

rss2html.com
<http://www.rss2html.com/>

rss2html.php
<http://www.feedforall.com/more-php.htm>

SimplePie
<http://simplepie.org/>

zFeeder
<http://zvonnews.sourceforge.net/zfeeder.php>

APPENDIX C

Feed Filtering and Mashing Tools

BlogSieve (mashing and/or filtering)
<http://www.blogsieve.com/>

FEEDblendr (mashing)
<http://feedblendr.com/>

FEEDcombine (mashing)
<http://www.feedcombine.co.uk/st/content/makefeed/>

FeedRinse (mashing and/or filtering)
<http://feedrinse.com/>

FeedShake (mashing and/or filtering)
<http://www.feedshake.com/>

FeedSifter (filtering)
<http://feedsifter.com/>

P.O.D. Principles:
Producing, Organizing,
and Distributing Podcasts
in Health Sciences Libraries and Education

Nadine Ellero
Ryan Looney
Bart Ragon

SUMMARY. With the integration of iPods and other mobile devices, podcasting has emerged as a potentially disruptive technology. Libraries are striving to discern what is appropriate when it comes to the production or distribution of podcasts. Many libraries are organizing podcast resources, some are producing their own content, and others are enabling their users to produce their own. These complex issues lead to difficult questions such as should this new medium be cataloged and how. doi:10.1300/J115v26S01_05 *[Article copies available for a fee from The Haworth Document Delivery Service: 1-800-HAWORTH. E-mail address: <docdelivery@haworthpress.com> Website: <http://www.HaworthPress.com> © 2007 by The Haworth Press, Inc. All rights reserved.]*

Nadine Ellero, MLS, AHIP (npe6f@virginia.edu) is Intellectual Access Librarian; Ryan Looney, MAS, MEd (rpr3u@virginia.edu) is Educational Technology and Research Coordinator; and Bart Ragon, MLIS (bart@virginia.edu) is Assistant Director for Library Technology Services and Development; all at the Claude Moore Health Sciences Library, University of Virginia, PO Box 800722, Charlottesville, VA 22908.

[Haworth co-indexing entry note]: "P.O.D. Principles: Producing, Organizing, and Distributing Podcasts in Health Sciences Libraries and Education." Ellero, Nadine, Ryan Looney, and Bart Ragon. Co-published simultaneously in *Medical Reference Services Quarterly* (The Haworth Information Press, an imprint of The Haworth Press, Inc.) Vol. 26, Supp. #1, 2007, pp. 69-90; and: *Medical Librarian 2.0: Use of Web 2.0 Technologies in Reference Services* (ed: M. Sandra Wood) The Haworth Information Press, an imprint of The Haworth Press, Inc., 2007, pp. 69-90. Single or multiple copies of this article are available for a fee from The Haworth Document Delivery Service [1-800-HAWORTH, 9:00 a.m. - 5:00 p.m. (EST). E-mail address: docdelivery@haworthpress.com].

Available online at http://mrsq.haworthpress.com
© 2007 by The Haworth Press, Inc. All rights reserved.
doi:10.1300/J115v26S01_05

KEYWORDS. Podcasts, podcasting, cataloging, lectures, libraries, medical libraries, sound recording, audio recording, course instruction, mobile devices, RSS feeds, portable devices, portable computerized instruments

OVERVIEW

Podcast is a term that many people associate with audio files that are downloaded from the Internet and played back on a mobile device, such as an iPod. This description is true, but doesn't capture the essence of what makes podcasting an innovation above and beyond merely creating and sharing digital content. A podcast can actually be one of several types of multimedia files and may be played on any device with the appropriate software, including iPods, other mobile audio and video players, as well as desktop and laptop computers. The "gee whiz" factor of a podcast comes not from the multimedia file, but rather from the code associated with the file that allows specialized software to automatically download new podcast episodes.[1] RSS syndication makes it possible for software like iTunes to seek out new content and deliver it to the user automatically.

Adding podcasts to any repertoire has several advantages. With a device such as an iPod, podcasts are portable. Podcasts, whether video, audio, or enhanced audio, offer another mode of content distribution. Podcasts allow institutions to capture and distribute archival content, such as lecture series. Patrons, especially those in the "21st Century Learner" demographic, are already incorporating podcasts into their routines, so offering podcasts is a way to meet them where they are.

PODCASTING PROCESS

The process for podcasting is relatively simple. An audio or video file is placed on the Web and referenced by an RSS (Really Simple Syndication) file. RSS syndication makes it possible for software like iTunes to seek out new content and deliver it to the user automatically. However, for many librarians, this can appear to be a daunting task since many of them may have never entered into the complex world of audio-video editing, compression, and XML. To add to this trepidation, podcasting is a relatively new technology, so many of the terms are new to librarians and not formally standardized even among the information technology community.

Before creating a podcast, it is advantageous to first understand how a podcast series works. A few simple concepts are true whether speaking of audio or video podcasts. Podcasts can be thought of in a similar fashion to a television series. The television series occurs over a period of time, and within the series there are individual episodes. A podcast series operates in much the same way. For example, there might be a library podcast series that provides instructional vignettes on searching PubMed. Each vignette is analogous to a television episode.

The podcast is organized and presented to the user via a form of XML known as RSS. RSS is the underlying technology for blogs, and in fact, podcasts were originally known as audioblogs. RSS files have two distinct sections: channel and item. The channel section contains metadata that describes the series. Table 1 is based on examples from the Technology at Harvard Law RSS 2.0 Specification document, which is an excellent source for learning about RSS.[2] For the purposes of this article, the examples and descriptions have been changed in Table 1 to be more appropriate for medical librarians.[3]

In addition to these tags, several optional tags help make the podcast feeds more usable for computer applications to interpret and repurpose. Examples of optional tags include category, docs, image, and lastBuildDate. Individual libraries creating podcasts should determine what data are most likely to be usable today and into the future. It is important to note that all of the channel tags are descriptive of the podcast series and not the individual items (or episodes).

All tags for items are optional in the sense that none are required for the RSS file to validate; however, there will need to be at least one title or description tag per item, and the enclosure tag referencing the audio or video file is needed so that the podcast will work. Table 2 represents a list of elements recommended by the authors.

In addition to the channel and item tags, libraries may wish to consider using the iTunes tags. iTunes has made huge gains in market share

TABLE 1. RSS Series Tags

Element	Description	Example
Title	This is the name of the podcast series.	Pubmed short courses
Link	Link to the Web site where the podcast exists.	http://www.your_url_here.com
Description	Abstract describing the scope and content of the series.	Learn the latest tips and tricks for using Pubmed.

TABLE 2. Item RSS Tags

Element	Description	Example
title	The title of the item (or episode)	<title>Exporting Pubmed Citations to Endnote.</title>
link	Link to the Web page for the item.	<link>http://www.your_url_here.com/ 215.html</link>
description	An abstract of the item.	<description>The following vodcast will provide basic instruction on importing Pubmed citations into Endnote. </description>
author	Speaker(s) and/or presenters.	<author>Joe Endnote</author>
category	Keywords or categories that best describe the episode.	< category>Endnote, Pubmed, exporting citations</category>
enclosure	Reference to the location of the audio or video file.	<enclosure url="http:// www.your_url_here.com /moviename.mp4" length="1024" type="video/mov"/>
guid	Global Unique Identifier. In many cases this may be the same as the link tag. However, this provides a unique identifier that can be referenced for cataloging.	<guid>http://www.your_url_here.com/ 215.html</guid>
pubDate	Date podcast was published.	<pubDate>Thu, 7 Sep 2006 09:50:12 -0400</pubDate>

as an audio/video player.[2] iTunes is also powerful as a directory and search engine for finding and downloading podcasts. The iTunes tags can be utilized by referencing the iTunes DTD (document type definition). A DTD is merely a document that defines what the iTunes tags are and how they can be used. Libraries need not worry about the technical details referenced in the DTD; rather, they should follow the instructions provided by Apple to properly use the tags.[4]

When considering the creation of a podcast, it is important to understand that content creation is most often the hardest part. To create a usable podcast a library must first define the scope and content of the podcast. Defining the scope will help establish the focus of the content that the library wishes to present. A podcast that meanders with no clear continuity will quickly lose users and fail to bring others back. Library news is an example of a potential podcast series whose subject matter shares a common scope. There are also other content areas that libraries can leverage to create useful podcasts for their users. One such example is a series of podcasts that teaches short educational vignettes, such as the PubMed example above. Since podcasting is still a relatively new concept, libraries, academic institutions, and third-party vendors are all working with this medium to try and leverage new services into high quality and usable products.

PODCASTING AND LIBRARIES

Although podcasting is new, there are perhaps three areas where libraries have seen significant growth in this technology. Marketing is one area where podcasting lends itself naturally for promoting library services and events. Many libraries now have tours up on the Web as podcasts, and some libraries have an iPod available for checkout for self-guided tours. Deborah Lee, in her article, "iPod, You-pod, We-pod, Podcasting and Marketing Library Services," states:

> Even the ubiquitous library tour could be developed with particular audiences in mind. In an academic environment, one podcast tour might be developed for the freshmen writing their first composition paper, another for graduate students at the dissertation stage, and yet another for new faculty on campus.[5]

In a health sciences or hospital library, developing specialized library podcast tours for medical students, residents, and other health professionals may not be the most effective use of time. However, Deborah's point of developing specialized content with a particular audience in mind is a valid one for a medical library setting. One library targeting a specific user group is the Health Sciences Library and Biocommunications Center at the University of Tennessee Health Science Center, which has created podcasts for students. "Designed for students on the go, the library podcasts are audio and video files that summarize highlights of library workshops and orientations that students can view in about 5 minutes or less."[6]

Podcasting provides libraries and other educational institutions with another route toward satisfying their educational and informational missions. When creating podcasts, using sound pedagogical principles provides the most effective results. Podcasting is inexpensive, and the technical aspects are relatively easy to master. However, podcasting should not be a catch-all technology, but rather another tool to be used to enhance learning, or to make available information or instruction that would otherwise not be available. Production of a podcast should be treated like any other piece of instruction. The desired learning outcomes and the needs and preferences of the target audience should be considered before production begins.

One way to start becoming more knowledgeable about podcasts, and more specifically, good quality podcasts, is to compile a list or directory of podcasts relevant for patrons. The Arizona Health Sciences Library maintains a list of medical podcasts that are pertinent to the needs of their patrons.[6] The process of finding and evaluating podcasts for inclusion on this type of list helps the staff to become more familiar with the technology of podcasting, as well as the potential uses for podcasting.

The easiest route to producing a podcast is to take existing content and put it into podcast format. Most libraries have instructional sessions and classes that might lend themselves to being recorded and made into a podcast. However, it's important to keep in mind how well a live event will translate into a podcast format. Podcasting an audio recording of a live, hands-on class may meet the goal of implementing online learning via a podcast, but it may not be useful to library patrons. During the class, the instructor may be moving about the room, answering students' questions, speaking extemporaneously, and visually leading the class through hands-on exercises and demonstrations. The interaction and dynamic nature that makes an in-person class interesting may make an audio (or even video) podcast difficult to follow, and unable to satisfy instructional objectives.

A better first step would be to consider a class or event that relies less heavily on student/teacher interaction, visuals, and hands-on experience. Lecture series are particularly well-suited to being podcast. Generally, the speaker is well-prepared and standing at a podium, making it easy to capture good-quality audio. A lecture is generally delivering informational content, rather than trying to teach psychomotor or cognitive skills. At the Claude Moore Health Sciences Library at the University of Virginia, the History of the Health Sciences lecture series is podcast.[7] These podcasts serve to preserve the lectures, making them available both for those who attended and those who, due to time or distance, were unable to attend. Making these podcasts available and searchable on iTunes allows them to reach a much wider audience than just the live lecture. Cataloging of these podcasts means their content is available for searching and use by students and researchers.

Podcasts can be incorporated into existing live classes, as supplemental materials. Various theories of learning styles, such as the VARK theory,[8] indicate that some people may learn information more readily when it is presented in an audio format. For those patrons that do prefer to learn aurally, a podcast can reach them in a way that printed materials can't, and the portability of podcasts fits in with students' busy life-styles. Many universities provide audio recordings of lectures for their students, and companies such as Apple realize the huge market that educational institutions represent. Apple has already created iTunes U, a service that allows for universities to place their content within the iTunes application and utilize all of its directory and searching features.[9] According to a recent article in the *Chronicle of Higher Education*, the University of California at Berkeley has been podcasting for over a year and has recently posted lectures from 30 courses within the iTunes framework.[10] This content is freely available to everyone within and outside of the university community. Obadiah Greenberg, the product manager for Berkeley's Webcasting services, was quoted in the article as saying, "We're reaching out to an entire worldwide community of self-learners . . . The walls of the ivory tower are coming down a bit."[10] The University of Michigan's School of Dentistry was one of the pilot programs for Apple's iTunes U. Students are able to subscribe to lectures and other course materials using a special portal within iTunes. Lectures being available for review after the class has ended means that students can use recordings of their professors, rather than relying on their own notes, to review the information presented. The value of these podcasts is not just in preserving lectures, but also in allowing them to be portable. When loaded onto a portable device, such as an iPod, students can now review lectures at their convenience, whether that is in their cars, at the gym, or at home. These audio-only podcasts allow a portability and integration into the lives of the students that other file types, such as video, can't offer. On-demand technologies, like podcasting, are becoming more and more ubiquitous, and are almost an expected part of an academic environment.

Academic podcasting isn't limited to iTunes U, or to recorded lectures. Purdue University hosts and syndicates its own materials, and creates material that is produced solely for the podcast format.[11] In this example, course materials were produced specifically for podcast format. They are supplements to in-class instruction and contain review of material taught in class, as well as introductions to future topics. Like the Michigan School of Dentistry podcasts, much of the value of these podcasts is in their portability. Students can listen to them while doing other things, rather than having to devote their full attention to printed material or a video.

Another potential use for podcasting in libraries is to offer instruction in podcasting to patrons. With free, user-friendly software like GarageBand (Macintosh) or Audacity (Macintosh and PC), nearly anyone can learn to podcast. The Claude Moore Health Sciences Library at the University of Virginia incorporated podcasting in the curriculum of its annual Multimedia Bootcamp.[12] Participants learn the basics of how podcasting works, then spend two intensive days scripting and producing their own podcasts. The technology to produce a podcast is relatively simple to master, and participants finish the program by demonstrating their completed podcasts. This type of educational programming serves to increase awareness of the technology services and support offered by the library. The course also supports the educational mission of the University by focusing on how to integrate technology into teaching.

Podcasting can also serve as a way to keep patrons up to date with library events, policies, hours, and other changing information. RSS allows for alerts to be pushed to a variety of containers, whether those containers are Web pages, e-mails, blogs, RSS readers, or other types of applications. Once users are subscribed to a podcast, they will automatically receive any new updates. They don't have to seek library information; library information comes to them. RSS and podcasting have flipped the idea of push technologies upside down. In the past, libraries would push alerts, updates, and news via e-mail, listervs, etc. RSS allows not only for the same information to be pushed in the same manner, but it allows for the other technologies to pull that same information. In other words, readers or aggregators–in the case of podcasts, known as podcatchers–can pull the information directly from the source. All that is needed is access to the RSS file. Every time the RSS file is updated, the podcatcher will pull the information to the location specified by the user. Users have totally embraced pull technologies. Mobile devices such as iPods and cell phones will become more integrated into everyday life when pull technologies become more prevalent and in demand.

For libraries just starting out, a brief podcast of library information is simple to produce. A short script, basic recording equipment, such as a microphone connected to a PC, and audio editing and conversion software such as Audacity or GarageBand are all that is required. Careful planning and scripting can result in a podcast that contains clear information relevant to patrons' needs.

Beyond audio library tours, libraries are using podcasts to disseminate a variety of information. Dowling College produces a monthly podcast that not only includes facts and information about the library, but also has interviews and human interest segments.[13] The journalistic piece of this podcast series serves as the hook, capturing patrons' attention and increasing interest in the library's podcast. Increased interest in this podcast means that more patrons are exposed to information about the library.

The Decatur Campus of Georgia Perimeter College produces a short monthly podcast with information about the library.[14] The Web page for these podcasts is a blog and uses this format as a companion to the podcasts. Each blog entry contains a link to the podcast, as well as links and resources that pertain to the content within the podcast. By pairing the blog with the podcast, GPC has made many pieces of information available to patrons, depending on their preferences. The podcast is short, but contains valuable information about the library. Each podcast/blog entry provides the opportunity to gather more information, if the user so desires.

The informational podcast can serve as a jumping-off point to more instructionally focused podcasts. Rather than being a supplement to class material, the "InfoPods" podcasts of the University of Buffalo Health Sciences Library are standalone instructional pieces <http://ublib.buffalo.edu/hsl/ref/mp3/>. They are designed from the ground up to take advantage of the audio podcast format, rather than adapting existing content to fit the tool.

In the area of health sciences and libraries there seems to be a lot of different directions. Health sciences and medical libraries seem to struggle with the decision of how to address explosive and even disruptive technologies. Since library patrons from the health professions tend to have busy lives, it is hard to decide what is an explosive and useful technology, and what is a fad. In addition, creating well constructed content for a podcast is time consuming. Many health sciences and medical libraries are just now beginning to evaluate the usefulness of podcasting library content to their patrons. However, health sciences and medical libraries have not been inactive. Many libraries have developed sites that categorize and organize podcast feeds from third-party vendors. Types of podcasts being made available include CME, consumer health, and table of contents.

No matter what a library decides to podcast, one thing is for certain; content is king. A library should make sure that it understands the commitment it is making with beginning a podcast series. It is not appropriate to decide to create a podcast series only to produce one or two and move on to other things. Once a library decides on the scope and focus of the content, it can turn its attention to establishing a good model handling the technical considerations of managing its content.

CREATING AND DISTRIBUTING PODCASTS

In terms of creating audio only content, there are several options. Audacity <http://audacity.sourceforge.net/> is an open source utility that is well developed and free to both the Windows and Mac platforms. It has a large community of developers with support for beginners as well as advanced users. Once Audacity is downloaded and installed, a microphone can be plugged into the computer to begin recording. On Audacity's Web site, there is a FAQ section, tutorials, documentation manuals, and a wiki. Beginners should take some time to review the information that is available to them as well as practice using the program before creating a production level audio file. Well thought out content should be storyboarded prior to beginning the podcast. In many cases, it is advantageous to create a script prior to the recording process. When possible, a speaker should be chosen who has a nice recording voice, and the speaker should speak with an even level and pleasant cadence. Once the podcast has been recorded, Audacity will save the project in an aup format, which is not readable by most audio players. The aup file is the working project file and should be saved in this format so that the project is editable at a later date. To produce Web-friendly formats, an mp3 file should be created. Mp3 offers some compression options that will make the podcast more consumable to podcatchers and audio players. At the Claude Moore Health Sciences Library, the "History of the Health Sciences" lecture series is podcast and most of the hits do not come from podcatchers, but from direct hits off of the Web site <http://www.healthsystem.virginia.edu/internet/library/historical/lectures.cfm>. For this reason, the Library tries to create a file size that is around 8 MB or smaller. Any time a file is compressed, there is some loss in quality. A balance needs to be achieved between compressing the file to a usable size, and not compressing so much that the audio file is of poor quality. The Library tested several methods of compression as well as consulted with audio experts in the University of Virginia community and settled on using the compression settings shown in Table 3.

TABLE 3. Compression

Compression Option	Compression Setting
sample rate	44 KHz
bit	16
Stereo/Mono	Mono

With these settings there is a noticeable loss of quality when comparing with the original file; however, the loss in quality is not so great that it distracts from the podcast. Any higher compression produced an audio file that sounded like it was recorded in a tunnel, and any lower compression produced a file that was too large.

Prior to creating the mp3 file, some editing may need to be done. For example, in the case of the lecture series, the speaker may have high or low audio spikes based on the speaker's intonation. Audacity allows for the manual editing of these peaks and valleys in the audio file so that it can be created as a more even podcast. There are also programs such as Levelator <http://www.gigavox.com/levelator/> that can compress, normalize, and limit an audio file automatically. Levelator is free and can be a useful utility; however, users will want to check the audio file to ensure that quality standards are maintained.

If archiving the podcast is a concern, a wav file should be produced. A wav file compressed at 44 KHz and 16 bit is considered CD quality, and will ensure that a high quality audio file can always be created in the future. Next, the mp3 file can be created. Audacity does not have the built-in ability to export to mp3. However, there is a freely available LAME MP3 encoder on the Audacity Web site <http://audacity.sourceforge.net/help/faq?s=install&item=lame-mp3>. Once this encoder is downloaded and installed, Audacity can be used to export into mp3 format. The export process will present the user with the ID3 options. ID3 tags are a form of metadata that is associated with the audio file itself. This includes information like artist, album, year, and genre. Windows users will see this information if they download the file directly to their hard drive and use Windows Explorer to locate the file. OSX users will see this information in the Get Info dialog box. Most media players will also display portions of this information. Table 4 is an example using version 2 of the ID3 tags.

After the mp3 file is produced, the audio file can be placed on a Web accessible server and then the RSS file created, as described previously. Since RSS is a form of XML, the rules of XML apply. XML standardizes what fields are optional and what fields are required. Often there are restrictions to the formatting of data contained within the tags, such as publication date. This ensures that the data are consistent and usable for ancillary applications. For this reason, it is recommended that podcast creators validate their RSS file. Web sites such as Feed Validator <http://feedvalidator.org/> will do this free of charge. After placing the RSS file in a Web accessible location, a pointer must be created to its Web location, and Feed Validator will check the code. If there are any

TABLE 4. ID3 Tags

ID3v2 Tag	Description	Example
Title	Title of the lecture	The Last Days of the Iron Lung
Artist	Speaker's name	Dudley F. Rochester, M.D.
Album	Podcast Series	The History of the Health Sciences Lecture Series, Claude Moore Health Sciences Library, UVA
Track Number	The lecture number in the year's sequence	2
Year	The year recorded	2005
Genre		speech
Comments	Any additional comments	leave blank

elements that do not validate, Feed Validator will highlight the code and provide some basic troubleshooting information and documentation. Once the RSS file has been validated, a library can then direct users to this file for use with their podcatcher. However, podcast producers may want to consider using services such as FeedBurner <http://www. feedburner.com>. FeedBurner is a free service that provides three major advantages to podcasters. First, it reads the RSS file and then provides a separate Web address that formats the XML code into a Web page that is readable to end users and is subscribeable to podcatchers. Second, it provides a link that will launch the default media player on end users' computers. Lastly, since podcasters can edit their accounts, it provides a stable URL. Should podcasters ever need to change the location of their RSS file, they can update this information within FeedBurner, and pod-catchers will continue to be able to access the RSS file with no change from the end user.

There are two additional types of podcasts that can be created. Enhanced audio podcasts are podcasts that can contain images and links that are associated with the audio file. Enhanced audio podcasts can be created using the Mac application Garage Band or by following the PodcastChapterTool located on the voxmedia wiki <http://www. voxmedia.org/wiki/PodcastChapterTool>. These images are then displayed in a slideshow format that can be seen on many iPods and within iTunes. Podcast creators should be mindful that many applications such as RealPlayer cannot play this format. Video podcasts, or vodcasts, are becoming more prevalent as this technology grows in popularity. Creating video involves many of the same issues as creating an audio podcast, including content creation; editing, and compression. Video can often be more time consuming to create, edit, and revise. Libraries should consider the time investment and sustainability of the content prior to production and note that vodcasts can uniquely captivate and engage users. Additional equipment and considerations such as a digital video camera and lighting will need to be considered. More extensive information on how to vodcast can be found at Wikipedia <http://en.wikipedia.org/wiki/Video_podcast> and Playlist <http://playlistmag.com/features/2005/07/howtovodcast/index.php>.

THE QUESTION OF CATALOGING

Podcasts are new channels leading users to new content, and at the Claude Moore Health Sciences Library, a cataloging opportunity presented itself when the "History of the Health Sciences Lecture Series" ceased analog form (i.e., audiotapes and audiocassettes) and was refashioned in 2005 into audio digital files that were transmitted via a webcast which could be downloaded or accessed via podcast <http://www.healthsystem.virginia.edu/internet/library/historical/lectures.cfm>. The "History of the Health Sciences Lecture Series" is a unique series of lectures sponsored by the Library and the University of Virginia School of Medicine Continuing Medical Education Program each academic semester and held in the Wilhelm Moll Rare Book and Medical History Room on the ground floor of the Claude Moore Health Sciences Library. These lectures represent a spectrum of topics, such as "The Cloth Monkey and the Life of Harry Harlow" (Deborah Blum), "Discovering the Insulin Documents" (Dr. Michael Bliss), and "Last Days of the Iron Lung" (Dr. Dudley F. Rochester). All of these lectures feature well known professionals in their fields of expertise and have been cataloged for the past 24 years in OCLC (Online Computer Library Center) <http://www.oclc.org/> and the local OPAC (Online Public Access Catalog). Several staff at the Claude Moore Health Sciences Library and the University of Virginia Library met to discuss the feasibility of cataloging podcasts. These podcasts represented series that either had a history of cataloging by the libraries or were content-rich lectures given at the University and made available via a podcast. The consensus was to continue cataloging these newly created podcasts of guest lectures or class instructions as the catalog record/resource description (i.e., personal name entries, subjects, detailed summary fields) is a rich metadata source for resource discovery whether utilizing an OPAC, OCLC

WorldCat, or a universal search engine such as Yahoo or Google. Currently, it is challenging to effectively search podcasts when the specific title or speaker is unknown and a general search query is executed, such as "women in medical research ["and-ed" with] podcasts." Consider the searcher who is unaware that a podcast of Gertrude Elion exists. Gertrude Elion was a 1988 Nobel Prize Winner and an excellent example of a woman in medical research. The goal in this case would be to facilitate discovery of the podcast interview of Gertrude Elion <http://invention.smithsonian.org/video/vids/pod_elionPt1.mp3> and <http://invention.smithsonian.org/video/vids/pod_elionPt2.mp3>. The MARC catalog record can contain additional information for resource discovery that goes beyond the speaker and lecture title. Medical Subject Headings, such as Biomedical Research, Research Personnel, Women, and Interviews, can be added to help facilitate a broader retrieval. The practice at the Claude Moore Health Sciences Library has been to include content-rich summaries, additional links to related Web resources, extensive subject analysis, and course learning objectives (see the 500 note on the Medical Center record in Figure 1).

To prove further the advantage of cataloging podcasts and not bypassing them as insignificant, the authors conducted a "Podcast Environmental Scan" in Health Sciences Libraries, in Other Academic Libraries, and in General Networks and Academic Medical Centers to determine how prevalent podcasts have become in the health sciences and general academic environments <http://www.people.virginia.edu/~npe6f/podcast/>. They found podcasting to be growing steadily and utilized for hosting five-minute updates or advertisements and presenting hour-long guest or course lectures. Mary Madden, author of the November 2006 Pew Internet & American Life Project on "Podcast Downloading," stated that, "The range of content available to those interested in podcasts has exploded over the past two years."[15] Podcasts offer quick publishing and are here until the next newest technology refashions them into a more optimal service, just as the audiocassette tape technology offered portability and served a better purpose over other recorded media, such as the LP (long playing record).

In addition to "The History of the Health Sciences Lecture Series," the Claude Moore Health Sciences Library held a long-standing practice of cataloging the "Medical Center Hour" series when it was first recorded on a physical medium. The "Medical Center Hour" began podcasting in 2005 and is another unique series of lectures hosted by the University of Virginia's Center for Humanism in Medicine <http://www.virginia.edu/uvapodcast/search.php?submit=true&filter=MedCenterHour>.

FIGURE 1. MARC Record of an Episode of the Medical Center Hour

Fixed Fields

Rec_Type	:g	Bib_Lvl	:m	Enc_Lvl	:I
Desc	:a	TypeCtrl	:	Entrd	:060615
Dat_Tp	:s	Date1	:2006	Date2	:
Ctry	:vau	Lang	:eng	Mod_Rec	:
Source	:d	Time	:060	Audience	:f
Accomp	:	GovtPub	:s	Type_Mat	:v
Tech	:l				

001		ocm70117478
003		OCoLC
005		20060615021159.0
007		vd cgaiz-
040		VAM|cVAM
090		R11|b.M4 2/8/2006
049		VAMB|c1|aVAMH|c2
245	00	How doctors think|h[videorecording] :|bclinical judgment and the practice of medicine /|c[presented by] the University of Virginia Medical School.
260		Charlottesville, Va. :|bThe University, [Clinical Engineering, Media Production Services],|cc2006.
300		1 videodisc (60 min.)|bsd., col. ;|c4 3/4 in. +|escript.
440	0	Medical center hour ;|v2/8/06
520		Kathryn Montgomery, Ph.D. (Professor of Medical Humanities and Bioethics, and of Medicine; Director,
		Medical Humanities and Bioethics Program, Northwestern University) described what she has observed as differences in the way doctors and scientists think. Among the aspects Dr. Montgomery explored were: case based reasoning (the narrative),
		the process of research and logic, medical education, evidence based medicine, and physician values and ethics.
538		DVD.
511		Panelists: Kathryn Montgomery, Daniel M. Becker; moderator, Julia E. Connelly.
500		Learning Objectives: 1. Discuss clinical judgment -- 2. Discuss the limits of the description of medicine as a science.
500		The Medical Center Hour is produced by The Center

FIGURE 1 (continued)

```
                    for Humanism in Medicine, University of Virginia
                    School of Medicine. The Medical Center Hour's
                    website is: http://www.healthsystem.virginia.
                    edu/internet/him/mch.cfm.
500                 "Medicine & Society in Conversation."
530                 Also available via webcast, download, or podcast as
                    viewed 9/19/2006.
650        2        Clinical Competence
650        2        Physician's Role
650        2        Thinking
650        2        Logic
650        2        Evidence-Based Medicine
650        2        Ethics, Medical
700        1        Montgomery, Kathryn,|d1939-
700        1        Becker, Daniel M.
700        1        Connelly, Julia E.
710        2        University of Virginia.|bSchool of Medicine.
856       41        |uhttp://www.virginia.edu/uvapodcast/popup.
php?submit=true&id=110


856       42        |3ACCESS TO GENERAL INFORMATION AND UPCOMING
SCHEDULE ONLY|uhttp://www.healthsystem.virginia.
edu/internet/him/
```

This weekly series held during the academic semester features topics intersecting medicine, the humanities, and the study of ethics. For cataloging purposes, the major difference between the "Medical Center Hour" and the "History of the Health Sciences Lecture Series" is that a physical DVD is produced in addition to the podcast for the "Medical Center Hour."

The cataloging question became an investigation of how to catalog within the confines of the MARC (Machine Readable Cataloging) structure. Admittedly, the MARC cataloging structure is not perfect or ideal, but it continues to populate the local OPAC and OCLC WorldCat databases. A more ideal environment would be to employ any and all structures that would allow resources to be effectively discovered regardless of venue used. The current wired/networked world demands more cooperation and integration. Trained catalogers/metadata specialists should be able to "directly" add, in real-time, enhanced metadata for resources wherever they reside, following cooperative models such as OCLC WorldCat and Wikipedia. This kind of intellectual access should be done once for the benefit of many throughout time.

MARC Cataloging Mechanics

MARC, while not as flexible or extensible as XML, does promote consistency and sharing of records within and among online catalogs. It is forecasted that a mass MARC conversion to XML or other XYZ structure will take place in the future, and while the time is not yet ripe for this large scale conversion, any current stretching of the MARC structure to accommodate new technology needs to be done with forethought and standardization in practices. The authors searched OCLC WorldCat to see if any podcasts had been cataloged and found that none had been cataloged as of September 2006, except for resources on or about podcasting and those added by the authors' library. In October 2006, the AUTOCAT listserv showed several postings seeking information on cataloging podcasts. As of this writing, there are no standard practices for cataloging podcasts, and the Claude Moore Health Sciences Library created its own standard, which is described later in this section. The main goal was to ensure retrieval with "podcast" as a limit. The word "podcast" needed to reside in a field that could be key word indexed and searched by the library's OPAC. Unfortunately, the 500 fields selected for the two different series are not, as of this writing, keyword indexed in OCLC WorldCat. The authors contacted OCLC regarding this lack of keyword indexing and OCLC responded by stating that they "are exploring the issue and would like to provide such capabilities in the future."[16]

The two unique podcast series described earlier in this paper required two slightly different cataloging practices. The "History of the Health Sciences Lecture Series" episodes, which solely exist as digital audio files, were cataloged using a sound recording record with file type "i," for "Nonmusical Sound Recording" with the fields listed in Table 5 illustrating the podcast features.

TABLE 5. MARC Fields and Values for "The History of the Health Sciences Lecture Series" Podcast

FIELD	CONTENT
245	|h [electronic resource]
300	1 audio file (52 min.) : |b digital, mono. + |e lecture flyer.
516	mp3 file available via webcast, download, or podcast.
856 40	|u http://www.virginia.edu/uvapodcast/popup.php?submit=true&id=136

Figure 2 is the full MARC record for "What's in a name?," the April 3, 2006 episode of the History of the Health Sciences Lecture Series.

On the other hand, the "Medical Center Hour" series, which has a physical form, was first cataloged as a DVD with the podcast added as

FIGURE 2. MARC Record of an Episode of the History of the Health Sciences Lecture Series

Fixed Fields

Rec_Type	:i	Bib_Lvl	:m	Enc_Lvl	:I		
Desc	:a	TypeCtrl	:	Entrd	:061026		
Dat_Tp	:s	Date1	:2006	Date2	:		
Ctry	:vau	Lang	:eng	Mod_Rec	:		
Source	:d	Comp	:uu	Format	:n		
Audience	:e	Repr	:s	Accomp	:z		
Ltxt	:hl						
TypeCode	:m	Frequn	:	Regulr	:		
Audience	:	FileType	:h	GovtPub	:		

001		ocm74470089
003		OCoLC
005		20061026031536.0
040		VAM|cVAM
090		R133.6|b.H4 4/3/2006
049		VAMB
100	1	Leavitt, Judith Walzer.
245	10	What's in a name?|h[electronic resource] : |bhistories of Mary Mallon and Typhoid Mary /|cJudith W. Leavitt.
260		Charlottesville, Va. :|bClaude Moore Health Sciences Library, University of Virginia Health System,|c2006.
300		1 audio file (52 min.) :|bdigital, mono. +|electure flyer.
440	0	History of the Health Sciences lecture series ;|v4/3/2006
440	0	Kenneth R. Crispell memorial lecture series.
500		The History of the Health Sciences Lecture Series is sponsored by the Claude Moore Health Sciences Library and the University of Virginia School of Medicine Continuing Medical Education Program as an educational service for the University of Virginia Health System and interested citizens in the community.

FIGURE 2 (continued)

```
516              mp3 file available via webcast, download, or
                 podcast.
500              Funded by the Wilhelm Moll Memorial Fund.
520              Judith W. Leavitt, Ph.D. (Rupple Bascon and Ruth
                 Bleier Wisconsin Alumni Research Foundation
                 Professor of Medical History, History of Science,
                 and Women's Studies, University of Wisconsin at
                 Madison) tells the story of the Irish cook Mary
                 Mallon, known as "Typhoid Mary, who was quarantined
                 against her will for 23 years." Dr. Leavitt
                 described how public health officials have often
                 protected the masses through the expense of
                 personal liberties. She showed how names can hurt
                 and change the course of a life, of history, of how
                 historians tell history and how stigmatizing names
                 can affect efforts to protect the public's health.
                 In addition, Dr. Leavitt revealed the woman behind
                 the caricature image, examined the power of
                 language/names through symbol and metaphor, and
                 outlined the many ways in which the complete
                 historical story matters for understanding, truth,
                 and present and future action.
500              Title from the lecture flyer.
500              "The tenth annual Kenneth R. Crispell Memorial
                 History Lecture." -- from program flyer.
600     10       Mallon, Mary.|
650     0        Stigma (Social psychology)
650     2        Typhoid Fever|xhistory|zUnited States
650     2        Public Health|xethics|zUnited States
650     2        Symbolism
650     2        Metaphor
650     2        Quarantine|xethics|zUnited States|
650     2        Quarantine|xhistory|zUnited States
710     2        Claude Moore Health Sciences Library.
856     40       |uhttp://www.virginia.edu/uvapodcast/popup.
php?submit=true&id=136
```

TABLE 6. MARC Fields and Values for "The Medical Center Hour" Podcast

FIELD	CONTENT
530	Also available via webcast, download, or podcast as viewed 9/19/2006.
856 41	|u http://www.virginia.edu/uvapodcast/popup.php?submit=true&id=303

an "additional format." Each episode has its own visual materials record with file type "g" for projected medium; Table 6 illustrates the fields used for the podcast features.

Figure 1 is the full MARC record for "How doctors think: clinical judgment and the practice of medicine," the February 8, 2006 episode of the Medical Center Hour.

CATALOGING SUMMARY AND CALL TO ACTION

Rick Anderson, Director of Resource Acquisition at the University of Nevada, Reno Libraries, stated that, "As a Web 2.0 reality continues to emerge, our users expect access to everything–digital collections of journals, books, blogs, podcasts, etc. You think they can't have everything? Think again. This may be our great opportunity."[17] New content and new channels will continue to evolve and become more efficient in performance, availability, and discoverability. Users will want everything now and delivered in ways that will facilitate better research and selection of resources. Would it not be more beneficial to retrieve a guidance page like that in Table 7 when searching "Gertrude Elion"?

New channels cannot cripple librarians' efforts at providing intellectual access, and perfect systems and tools will never be ready; yet, the effort must continue even with the less than ideal record structures and databases. Cataloging podcasts provided an opportunity to look at a new channel for content, to wrestle with the best ways to make these resources available in online Internet accessible catalogs, and to create a cataloging practice/standard where none existed. Colleagues were contacted and dialog was begun to hopefully create more energy for working cooperatively and encouraging the development of real-time tools tied to resources wherever they exist in space and time. Many institutions are creating valuable, rich information content channeled through podcasts. The call to catalog and preserve our institutions' creative memory and insure discoverability over time is the core responsibility of information management and the value that libraries add to parent institutions and the world.

TABLE 7. Simulated Future Search Engine Retrieval

Gertrude Elion–Biography [would include further division or search options by print, video or audio as well as by date] – Full Biography, Brief Biography, Interviews
Gertrude Elion–Lectures [would include further division or search options by print, video or audio as well as by date and subject]
Gertrude Elion–Research [would include further division or search options by print, video or audio as well as by date and subject]
Gertrude Elion–Writings [would include further division or search options by date and subject]
Gertrude Elion–Others like her; Contemporaries: Other Women in Biomedical Research, etc.

CONCLUSION

The technology to produce podcasts is easy to use, and the push/pull technology of disseminating them sets podcasting apart from merely creating and distributing multimedia content. Having good content is the best way to take advantage of the technology and requires some investment of time and effort. Useful content can take many different forms, and novel uses of podcasts are constantly being developed. Changes in end-user technology, such as portable audio/video devices and smartphones, can result in new ways of implementing podcasts. Creators of podcasts need only think outside of the box, always keeping the end user in mind. Cataloging podcasts is an important step in disseminating them. Podcasts are truly available to academia when they are treated like other parts of a library's collection.

REFERENCES

1. Podcast. Available: <http://en.wikipedia.org/wiki/Podcast>. Accessed: November 20, 2006.

2. "Technology at Harvard Law." Available: <http://blogs.law.harvard.edu/tech/rss>. Accessed: November 27, 2006.

3. "Apple's iTunes Player Climbs Streaming Media Charts–PC Time Tracks Broadband Penetration." Available: <http://www.websiteoptimization.com/bw/0603/>. Accessed: November 15, 2006.

4. "Podcasting and iTunes: Technical Specification." Available: <http://www.apple.com/itunes/store/podcaststechspecs.html>. Accessed: November 17, 2006.

5. Lee, Deborah. "iPod, You-pod, We-pod." *Library Administration & Management* 20(Fall 2006): 206-8.

6. "Medical Podcasts." Available: <http://www.ahsl.arizona.edu/weblinks/Medical_podcasts.cfm>. Accessed: November 20, 2006.

7. "UVa-HSL :: Lecture Series." Available: <http://www.healthsystem.virginia.edu/internet/library/historical/lectures.cfm>. Accessed: November 20, 2006.

8. Fleming, Neil. "VARK–A Guide to Learning Styles." Available: <http://www.vark-learn.com/english/index.asp>. Accessed: November 20, 2006.

9. "Apple–Education–Products–iTunes U." Available: <http://www.apple.com/education/products/ipod/itunes_u.html>. Accessed: November 17, 2006.

10. "Berkeley Offers Free Podcasts of Courses Through iTunes." *Chronicle of Higher Education*. 52(May 5, 2006): A44.

11. "BIOL 137 Rewind/Flash Forward Podcasts." Available: <http://www.bio.purdue.edu/mt/feeds/BIOL137/>. Accessed: November 20, 2006.

12. Looney, Ryan P., and Ramsey, Ellen C. "Multimedia Bootcamp: Encouraging Faculty to Integrate Technology in Teaching." *Medical Reference Services Quarterly* 25(Fall 2006): 87-92.

13. Kretz, Chris. "Learning to Speak: Creating a Library Podcast with a Unique Voice." Available: <http://www.higheredblogcon.com/index.php/learning-to-speak-creating-a-library-podcast-with-a-unique-voice/>. Accessed: November 20, 2006.

14. Free, David. "Listen Up!" Available: <http://gpclibraryradio.blogspot.com/>. Accessed: November 20, 2006.

15. Madden, M. "Podcast Downloading." Pew Internet & American Life Project (November 2006). Available: <http://www.pewinternet.org/pdfs/PIP_Podcasting.pdf>. Accessed: November 28, 2006.

16. de Gaia, Jamsine. E-mail, September 29, 2006.

17. Storey, T. "Web 2.0: Where Will the Next Generation Web Take Libraries?" *NextSpace* 2(2006): 7.

doi:10.1300/J115v26S01_05

Streams of Consciousness: Streaming Video in Health Sciences Libraries

Nancy T. Lombardo

Sharon E. Dennis

Derek Cowan

SUMMARY. Streaming media delivery on the Web has become a ubiquitous service expected by many of today's library patrons. Libraries can offer selection, preservation, dissemination, and production of streaming media content. The Spencer S. Eccles Health Sciences Library has offered its patrons streaming media and on-demand video services since 2000. A mobile video broadcasting unit was designed and implemented to

Nancy T. Lombardo, MLS (nancyl@lib.med.utah.edu) is Librarian, Spencer S. Eccles Health Sciences Library, University of Utah, 10 North 1900 East, Salt Lake City, UT 84112. She serves as the Systems Librarian, managing the Systems and Video departments at the library, as well as Principal Investigator on the Neuro-Ophthalmology Virtual Education Library, or NOVEL project.

Sharon E. Dennis, MS (sdennis@lib.med.utah.edu) is Librarian, Spencer S. Eccles Health Sciences Library, University of Utah, 10 North 1900 East, Salt Lake City, UT 84112. She serves as Technology Coordinator for the National Network of Libraries of Medicine (NN/LM) MidContinental Region (MCR) as well as Co-Director for the Health Education Assets Library (HEAL) multimedia database project.

Derek Cowan (dcowan@lib.med.utah.edu) is Digital Video Technician, Spencer S. Eccles Health Sciences Library, University of Utah, 10 North 1900 East, Salt Lake City, UT 84112. He manages the digital video studio and video services at the Eccles Library.

[Haworth co-indexing entry note]: "Streams of Consciousness: Streaming Video in Health Sciences Libraries." Lombardo, Nancy T., Sharon E. Dennis, and Derek Cowan. Co-published simultaneously in *Medical Reference Services Quarterly* (The Haworth Information Press, an imprint of The Haworth Press, Inc.) Vol. 26, Supp. #1, 2007, pp. 91-115; and: *Medical Librarian 2.0: Use of Web 2.0 Technologies in Reference Services* (ed: M. Sandra Wood) The Haworth Information Press, an imprint of The Haworth Press, Inc., 2007, pp. 91-115. Single or multiple copies of this article are available for a fee from The Haworth Document Delivery Service [1-800-HAWORTH, 9:00 a.m. - 5:00 p.m. (EST). E-mail address: docdelivery@haworthpress.com].

deliver live broadcasts of lectures and special events. Educational video digitization, production, and cataloging services were offered. Challenges and successes with this service are reported. doi:10.1300/J115v26S01_06 *[Article copies available for a fee from The Haworth Document Delivery Service: 1-800-HAWORTH. E–mail address: <docdelivery@haworthpress.com> Website: <http://www.HaworthPress. com>* © 2007 by The Haworth Press, Inc. All rights reserved.]

KEYWORDS. Streaming media, streaming video, on-demand video, library services

INTRODUCTION AND BACKGROUND

It is hard to believe that at the turn of this century, Internet users sat in excited anticipation for 20 minutes while downloading 30-second movie trailers, an enormous amount of time for possibly useless information. Today, streaming media is used to deliver all types of information. News media outlets use streaming video to bring a timely and realistic feel to their news reporting. Corporations use streaming video for corporate training and marketing. Entertainment venues promote their products through streaming video clips that widen their audience. Instructors deliver course material through streaming video over the Internet. Streaming video has become a ubiquitous and user friendly way to deliver information, educate, market services, and sell products.

Libraries must be involved at some level in order remain relevant to patrons. Informational video segments in all disciplines are now being offered for purchase or license, using streaming video as just another format. Many libraries are producing streaming video for a variety of patron services. Patrons have become accustomed to this type of information delivery. The library's role is to select, preserve, disseminate, and sometimes produce the best information sources available and make those accessible to patrons. Information collections and services must now include streaming video.

Many new issues and considerations come into play when including video streaming in the library's array of resources. All of the traditional considerations that libraries apply to acquisitions, collection development, access, archiving, and public services must be applied to streaming video, and new technologic and distribution issues may be required. The best video resources must be selected and evaluated, or created.

When appropriate, these resources must be indexed or cataloged, and patrons should be able to retrieve these resources when finding information. In some cases the video must be stored and made accessible. Video streaming can be time sensitive so may require agile and flexible capture and indexing procedures.

What Is Streaming Video?

Streaming video as a term is often used to describe any video that is delivered over the Internet. Technically, streaming video is not downloaded during play. The video is sent in a continuous stream of compressed information. The packets are buffered on the local hard drive, and then played by a client application on the local computer from the buffer. The video is essentially played as it arrives on the local computer, and the information is not retained on the hard drive. The user does need an appropriate client application, or player, but these are becoming more ubiquitous. Most computers come with at least one media player installed at time of purchase. The player application is able to read, uncompress, and display the video as it arrives over the network.

Major streaming video and streaming media applications include RealMedia Player from RealNetworks, Microsoft Windows Media Player, Apple's QuickTime Player, and Adobe's FlashPlayer. Additionally, many streaming video files are now embedded into the Web pages of the larger content sites and are viewed using browser plug-ins. Plug-ins are much easier to obtain and integrate today. In many cases, the delivery site can detect the lack of a specific plug-in and direct the user to download and install the plug-in in a matter of minutes, leading them directly back to the content.

The quantity and quality of streaming video received by the user are limited by the data rates of the connection (modem, ISDN, Cable, LAN, etc.). If the network connection is high bandwidth, the stream will perform well. When the network is congested, or if the connection is a low bandwidth modem, the stream may occasionally stall, or the image may be jerky or pixilated, displaying in blocks, and the audio may break up. As broadband access to the home has expanded in the United States, streaming media has become a standard information delivery mechanism.

Broadcast vs. On-Demand Streaming Video

Streaming is an excellent technology for both live event delivery and archival programming. A streaming broadcast, or webcast, refers to an event that is being recorded, streamed, and delivered live, as the event is taking place. This requires a streaming server, which takes the video signal as it is captured, converts it to a compressed streaming format, and sends that signal out over the Internet. A live broadcast is a synchronous event that must be viewed in real time, as the event is taking place. Like a radio or television program, the users connecting to a live stream will connect to the event as it is in progress. Users can connect at any time but will view the event from the point in time at which they make the connection. Archival programming, also called video on-demand, comprises those videos that have been recorded and stored on a video streaming server for later viewing. These streams are activated by the user and will be started at the beginning each time they are accessed by a remote user. This is asynchronous delivery, not dependent on time. Users get the entire stream delivered at their convenience, when they make the request by clicking on the activating link.

LITERATURE REVIEW

A review of the literature confirms that many libraries are using streaming video to enhance services and instruction. Many libraries are involved in video production to create library tours and instruction modules and support distance education, though there is not much evidence of libraries providing full-scale video broadcasting and production services to their patron communities, as is being done at the Spencer S. Eccles Health Sciences Library at the University of Utah.

An excellent overview of the history of video and the progression of its media is provided by Crow and Ondrusek.[1] Their point that librarians will be faced with new acquisition and delivery challenges due to the increasing availability of medical information in these new formats is important. Some popular information resources, such as the Bates' *Guide to Physical Examination* and the National Continuing Medical Education programming, are being made available in streaming video format. Licenses for these resources must be negotiated, as are the electronic journal and textbook resources today. Students and faculty must be educated in how to access the new formats from both on campus and remote locations. Additionally, some of these resources require local hosting, a technical service many health sciences libraries are not prepared to provide.

Large collections of content are starting to appear on the market, though they generally cover subject areas more relevant to undergraduate or

K-12 markets than to academic health sciences or hospital libraries. Nice reviews of some existing sources of content for more general use are provided in the three articles by Brown,[2] Ross,[3] and Valenza.[4] These articles also make clear the enthusiasm for streaming media by K-12 librarians. The delivery, budget, and student learning issues addressed by these authors are relevant to all libraries considering adding streaming media to their collections.

For libraries wanting to learn about the production process, a number of articles provide step-by-step instructions, suggestions, and recommendations for creating video resources. Two articles, by Hickok[5] and by Lee and Burrell,[6] present a well organized outline of the planning, production, and technical requirements involved when they created library instruction modules using streaming video. While many of the prices have lowered since these two experiences, the steps, planning, and process remain the same. Both of these articles describe the production of library instruction modules where the outcomes were positive and the benefits perceived to be well worth the effort. Crowther and Wallace[7] offer another good overview of the process, with less detail, but good suggestions for those getting started. These authors emphasize the value of streaming media for distance students. Cox and Pratt[8] focused on library instruction for remote users to serve the growing needs of their commuter students, as well as their distance education programs. They provide a good overview of their entire production process and positive reception by the users. Another positive experiment was described by Maness,[9] who created streaming video units to teach information literacy to engineering students. This author reports that the students surveyed indicated "similar rates of satisfaction, similar learning outcomes" and generally expressed acceptance of this mode of information delivery.

Some literature is available to describe use of screen capture tools to produce library instruction that can be delivered through streaming media. Templeman-Kluit and Eherenberg[10] describe why they chose to use screen capture. This team performed usability studies to help them determine the appropriate length and delivery factors. The screen capture production techniques proved most effective for the audience they planned to reach. Xiao, Pietraszewski, and Goodwin[11] describe in detail how they produced database instruction modules using screen capture technology. They also explain their rationale for selecting the technique.

Professional development for librarians is now regularly provided through streaming media. The College of DuPage programming for librarians is probably the best known and has been very successful in offering continuing education to librarians around the country. Joseph Barillari,[12] the Director of Information Technology Special Services and Manager of the Library Learning Network at the College of DuPage, describes the technology as "robust technically and popular with audiences," as well as cost effective, in his short article. The Medical Library Association Webcasts[13] for continuing education are delivered via streaming media. Stephen Abram,[14] President-elect of Special Libraries Association (SLA), advocates the use of streaming media and encourages librarians to learn more about it. He notes that it is being used by SLA for continuing education programming and is also used by Sirsi/Dynix for both internal and external training.

The two most prominent uses of streaming video by libraries are to provide library instruction to remote users and to provide continuing professional education to librarians. The majority of the literature indicates that this is a successful medium for these uses.

DELIVERING STREAMING MEDIA: SOFTWARE AND HARDWARE

Delivery Methods

Video and audio can be accessed on the Internet through two methods: as a streaming media file or as a downloaded media file.

Streaming media technology sends data continuously through the network, allowing the user to begin watching the file immediately and to continue watching it as it arrives; it simulates "real time" viewing of a video. An application on the server side transmits the streamed data; the user receives the data through a client application. The user can begin watching or listening to the streaming media file as soon as the receiving application has enough data to begin playing the file. Streaming media can be delivered in real-time (i.e., as a live broadcast, which the user can view as the event is happening) or on-demand (available for the user to access at any time, regardless of when the event took place). Live broadcasts may also allow some mechanism for interaction (for instance, asking questions of a speaker by phone or chat). If a streaming video is set up as a live broadcast, it can be recorded and offered on-demand for viewing at a later date.

Media files may also be available as simple downloads. This technology requires the user to download the entire video file before beginning to watch; if the file is large, this could take many hours. A hybrid method called progressive downloading allows the user to begin watching the video as soon as the file begins to download. The major advantage of the streaming format is that it allows the user to jump to any point in the video at any time, whereas progressive download forces the user to wait until the content has been received to move to a particular part of the video.

Delivery of streaming video requires a specialized video server. Users receiving the streaming video need to install appropriate client software, depending on the file format of the streaming video.

Streaming Media File Formats

Streaming media can be delivered in a variety of file formats. Some formats are suitable for streaming as a live broadcast and/or on-demand video; others are mostly used for on-demand video using the progressive download technique. The most commonly used formats are:

- Windows Media: content is delivered by streaming media as a live broadcast or on-demand archive.
- RealMedia: content is delivered by streaming media as a live broadcast or on-demand archive.
- QuickTime: content is generally delivered as an on-demand media file using progressive download.
- MPEG4: the MPEG4 format is a cross client format, and can be delivered to any media player.
- Macromedia Flash: content is generally delivered as an on-demand media file using progressive download.

Factors which potential streaming media producers must consider when choosing a delivery format include:

- Access to, or purchase of, the relevant server software, including costs, bandwidth availability, and system support.
- Access to the appropriate client software by the intended audience; willingness of the audience to download Web browser plug-ins or client software to support the media.
- Hardware preferences by the intended audience (for instance, an audience with Macintosh computers may prefer the QuickTime format, since Apple no longer supports the latest version of the Windows Media player).
- Expected future market share of the streaming media formats.

Streaming Media Servers and Clients

Libraries that wish to produce streaming media can purchase either a standalone server machine or a streaming server software package to be installed on an existing Web server. Streaming media software is available for all common server platforms such as Linux, Windows, etc.

Commonly available streaming media server software is listed below:

- Helix Universal Server from RealNetworks[15]: runs on the Windows and Linux operating system; formats supported include RealMedia, QuickTime, and MPEG-4. The cost is based on the amount of bandwidth used by the server. A 4 Megabits per second bandwidth license costs $2,000.00 with an annual support fee of $638.00 per year.
- Microsoft Windows Server 2003,[16] with the built-in Windows Media Server component: libraries with an existing Windows Server 2003 machine can install the Windows Media Server component to serve streaming media files without additional cost.
- Apple QuickTime Streaming Server[17] (QTSS): runs on the Macintosh OS X operating system; formats supported include QuickTime and MPEG4. QTSS is included as part of the Macintosh OS X Server software and costs $999.00 for an unlimited license.
- Darwin[18]: a free open source streaming media server for the Windows, Linux, and Solaris operating systems. Supported formats include QuickTime and MPEG-4. Although the code for Darwin is based on the commercial Apple QuickTime streaming server, it lacks a number of administrative and management features of QTSS. Technical support is not provided by Apple; developers must obtain support from the open source community.
- Adobe Flash Media 2[19]: runs on the Windows and Linux operating systems and supports the Adobe Flash format. It supports media files developed with the Flash authoring system, so it can support rich, interactive media applications in addition to delivering video. The server costs $4,500.
- It is also possible to stream media by purchasing space with an online hosting service; this eliminates the need to maintain an in-house server. Horizon Wimba[20] is an example of an online media hosting service.

Client software is usually offered as a Web browser plug-in or stand-alone application. The most basic version of the client software is available for free. Versions with more advanced features or subscription services are available for a small fee. Commonly used streaming media players include:

- RealPlayer.[21] The free player is still available but can be difficult to find on Real's Web site.
- Windows Media Player.[22] The Windows Media player is shipped with computers running the Windows operating system.
- QuickTime Player.[23]
- Flash Player.[24]

The formats that each player will support on installation are listed below. Most players will support other formats if appropriate plug-ins are installed.

RealPlayer: RealMedia, WindowsMedia, QuickTime, MPEG4, H.264
WindowsMedia Player: WindowsMedia, MPEG4, H.264
QuickTime: QuickTime MOV format, MPEG4, H.264
FlashPlayer: Flash video, SWF

Encoding Streaming Media Files

Delivering a video file through the Internet requires an enormous amount of bandwidth. Uncompressed video files are too large to send over the Internet; for instance, a full hour of taped footage in DV format is 12 gigabytes and will require 25 Megabits per second of bandwidth. To calculate the amount of bandwidth needed for any particular video, the size of the video frame (height and width) is multiplied by the frame rate (the number of frames or images that are projected or displayed per second). The formula for calculating bandwidth is:

frame height × frame width × frame rate (fps) = total bits/sec

As an example, a video with a height of 320, a width of 240 and 30 frames per second would require 2.3 Megabits per second of bandwidth (320 × 240 × 30 fps = 2.3 Mbps). A useful video bandwidth estimator is available on the Web.[25]

Videos are normally compressed in order for it to be viable to send them over the Internet. The videos are compressed using a software program called a codec (compression-decompression). The choice of a codec will depend upon a combination of factors: image quality, file size after compression, usability, and compatibility with the video server and client software.[26] A compressed streaming media file can be up to 100 times smaller than the original uncompressed file.

Codecs use a "lossy" compression scheme, meaning that large amounts of data are discarded during the compression process. The media files are decoded and decompressed on the fly by the player software, but the lost information is lost forever. Codecs try to reduce the amount of artifacts resulting from the lost data (fuzzy video, distortion in the audio or video, etc.). Codecs compress files by manipulating video variables (color depth, frame rate, window size, and degree of compression) and audio variables (audio bit rate, stereo or mono channels, and degree of compression).[27]

The Eccles Library generally encodes its streaming videos for live broadcast and archiving using the RealMedia codec included with the RealProducer software. Videos are encoded at 320 × 240 and 30 frames a second, with an audio bit rate of 22 Kbps mono. This produces an acceptable audio and video quality and can be viewed by users using a wide range of connection speeds, from 56k modems to T-1 lines. At the present time, the server software allows transmission of a video at a higher resolution, but users do not have the bandwidth to receive the signal.

To further accommodate users with different connection speeds, the stream can be broadcast at multiple bandwidth rates. The RealMedia Helix server uses a technology called SureStream to adjust the bandwidth of the stream to the actual connection speed of the user (see Figure 1).

Video and audio quality is a concern when delivering streaming media. Generally, users require higher quality audio and are more willing to tolerate lower quality videos. Minimizing extreme movements will reduce the amount of bandwidth used by the video.

If the video includes computer output such as PowerPoint display, it is important for the PowerPoint to have a large font size with a minimum of information on each slide. Screen shots or other intricate information will not display well on a 320 × 240 streaming video. The authors have found that this quality is good enough for most academic lectures that use PowerPoint, images, or videos as well as for panel discussions. It is not useful in a training session where a speaker needs to show software or Web site demonstrations.

Videos which are encoded and broadcast in real time, and then placed on the server for on-demand viewing, are left "as is" and not edited for quality. While it is possible to do post-processing to improve the quality, the volume of events being broadcast by the small number of staff at the Eccles Library makes it impossible to conduct post-production work on the videos. In some cases, the video is also saved in a raw format and

FIGURE 1. RealMedia SureStream Technology
<http://service.real.com/help/library/guides/ProductionGuide/prodguide/
htmfiles/realsys.htm#64854>

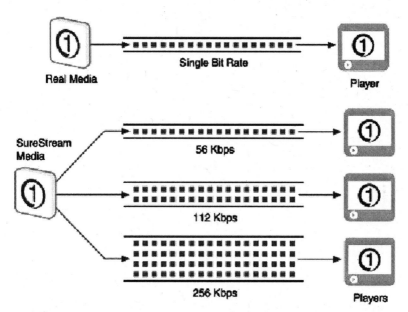

then edited and compressed into a streaming format, but these are the exception rather than the rule.

While users expect that academic lectures or classes will require the same amount of time to view as attending the event, usability experts recommend that the length of on-demand training videos be kept to a minimum. Nielsen conducted eye-tracking studies to find out which elements of the video frame users focused on during replay. He suggests that videos should not be more than a minute long, use video only when it is appropriate for the content, and avoid distracting elements.[28]

Hardware: The Mobile Unit

In order to facilitate the delivery of live broadcasts from a variety of locations at the Health Sciences Center, one of the authors (DC) designed a mobile video broadcasting unit. The unit consisted of modular components that could be swapped out or replaced in the event of equipment failure. It was stored in a large case on wheels to allow it to be quickly moved from one place to another.

The original unit was large (34″ × 25″ × 25″) and weighed over 200 pounds. It worked well for events within the Health Sciences Center but proved too unwieldy to ship to other locations for off-campus events (see Figure 2). A second "mini" unit was designed that is much smaller: it is closer to a suitcase size (21″ × 18″ × 16″) and weighs less than 40 pounds (see Figure 3). Both units are in daily use by the video studio staff, but the mini unit is used for off-campus events (see Figure 4).

Both mobile units consist of the following equipment:

Sturdy hard-shelled case: The case is one normally used by musicians to ship equipment from one place to another. The mini-unit case has foam insets to protect the equipment.

Camera and tripod: The large unit uses a TV production quality camera, Canon XL1. The mini unit uses a prosumer digital camera, the

FIGURE 2. Eccles Library's Original Mobile Unit

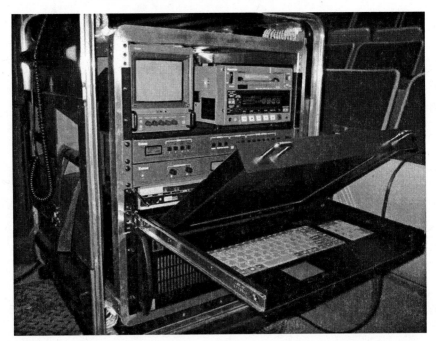

FIGURE 3. Eccles Library's Mini-Mobile Unit

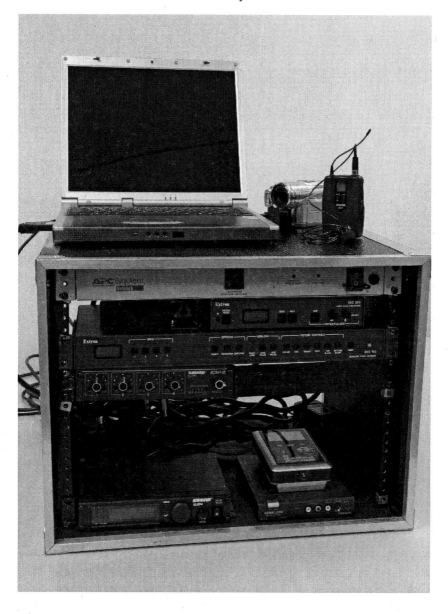

FIGURE 4. Complete Mobile Unit Comparison

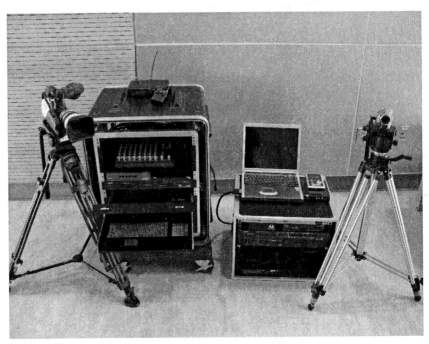

Panasonic PV-GS200. The large camera was appropriate for technicians with a lot of experience with video recording settings. The smaller camera has an automated mode that works well for less experienced librarians or technicians who are not familiar with video camera settings.

Computer and video capture card: The larger unit uses a desktop computer with full-size keyboard; the video capture card is built into the desktop. The mini unit has a laptop computer with an external bus to hold the Osprey 230 video capture card.

Scan converter: Many events feature a presenter who is using a computer to display a PowerPoint slide show or other computer output. The scan converter converts the digital signal from the presenter's computer to video format. Although it is possible to point the camera at the presentation screen, the quality of the resulting video is not as high as when the scan converter is used to convert the information.

Switcher: The switcher receives input from any number of sources, including the camera (for video) and the computer (for PowerPoint slides or other computer output). It then outputs the signal to the video capture card.

Audio equipment: The audio equipment consists of wireless microphones, wireless microphone receivers, and an audio mixer. The wireless microphone is worn by the speaker and makes it convenient for the speaker to move around the room; it sends a signal to the wireless microphone receiver. The audio mixer modulates the audio levels; it receives input from the receiver and outputs the audio the capture card. The broadcast technician can adjust the audio levels as needed during the presentation using the mixer.

Lighting: To keep the unit streamlined and easy to use, a lighting component was not added. While not usually an issue at the University of Utah Health Sciences Center, this can be an problem in other remote settings; in those cases, arrangements are made for local lighting equipment to be brought onsite.

DIGITAL VIDEO
AT THE ECCLES HEALTH SCIENCES LIBRARY

The Spencer S. Eccles Health Sciences Library at the University of Utah has been providing video production and delivery services to the Health Sciences Center since the year 2000. The service has been well utilized and has grown dramatically since its inception. Initially, there was a steep learning curve and lessons were learned the hard way at every live event. The Eccles Library offers broadcasting, archiving, and conversions services. As the "last mile" bandwidth has improved, providing more home users with high speed Internet connections, the use of streaming media for distance education courses has grown significantly.

The Eccles Library experience concurs with the findings of Adams[29] in his analysis of 409 distance education Web sites. His conclusion was that distance education programs are using streaming media, but not in a systematic way. The use of the technology at most distance education sites in his analysis appeared to be at the discretion of the faculty and was not selected based on research in instructional technologies or pedagogical need. The Eccles Library video services for distance education course lecture and seminar delivery has grown dramatically as the demand for distance education and the expectation for faculty to accommodate distance students has increased on this campus. Anecdotal evidence indicates that students prefer streaming media to previous methods, including the delivery of audio cassette tapes through U.S. mail, but the choice to employ streaming video seems to be based primarily on the fact that the service is free and available through the library, rather than on careful needs assessment of students or faculty.

As use of the video service has grown, the library has instituted a first come, first served policy, with priority always given to curriculum-related uses. Much of the current equipment used has been purchased through the library's allocation of student computing fees, so non-curriculum related projects that can be accommodated are also assessed a small fee to cover the cost. Conversion projects are subject to these same policies. Video can be converted for faculty teaching in the curriculum of the health sciences programs, but must be requested well ahead of the use date and are prioritized in the work flow after live or archived course lecture and seminar delivery projects.

History of Digital Video at Eccles Library: The Learning Curve

In January of 2000, the Eccles Health Sciences Library first implemented a digital video studio that would allow the library to provide conversion, broadcast, and archival production services to library patrons. Serving an academic health sciences center, there were many known potential applications. The University of Utah's School of Medicine has outlying clinics that would benefit from live broadcasts of seminars and medical rounds. The College of Nursing was expanding its distance education programming to meet the needs of students throughout the large rural region surrounding the Salt Lake City metropolitan area. These students would benefit from live broadcast and archived classroom lectures and seminars. The Medical Informatics program at the University of Utah was interested in broadcasting their weekly seminars. The Eccles Health Sciences Library hosts many special topic events and lectures that would benefit from expanded access through broadcast to the larger library and academic community. The possibilities seemed endless.

By piecing together a number of foundation gifts and grants, the library was able to purchase the necessary equipment. The library hired a consultant to prepare a list of recommended hardware and to provide some elemental training. At that time, the complete studio configuration cost $25,000.00. Initially, the studio worked with the MPEG1/2 video format using crude, hardware based encoding techniques. At that point in time, the quality was great, but files were huge. Outside the building, other sites on campus had problems viewing the video. Off-campus sites found it impossible to receive a viewable stream. The bandwidth requirements were enormous and it simply was not appropriate for the widely varied bandwidth speeds represented by the users' connections.

This caused the library to change focus and experiment with the RealMedia video format for live broadcasts. RealNetworks was the most accessible vendor for a broad audience at that date. The player was widely available and was free, which was an important consideration for library users. The RealMedia software suite allowed the library to broadcast live streams and easily archive video for on-demand playback. Both the live broadcasts and the archives were streamed over the Internet, meaning they begin to play quickly, without the user having to download the file to their computer. The ability to create "SureStreams" which can detect and accommodate a variety of bandwidths was attractive to the library, as the intended audience could range from faculty, staff, or students in the library's computer labs with high speed Internet connections to patrons in rural areas of the state with modem connections.

The initial server purchased to host the RealMedia software suite was a Dell PowerEdge 1300 with dual Pentium III 500MHz processors, 256MB of RAM, an Osprey video capture card, and 18GB storage. The system ran on Windows NT server software and hosted the RealServer and RealProducer. At the time, it was big, fast, and powerful. This machine was to be the mobile server, to be moved around to various locations for live broadcasting and immediate archiving. The digital video camera was a Canon XL1, and sound was captured with a Shure wireless remote microphone.

The staff of the digital video studio consisted of two personnel, the Systems Librarian and a Video Technician. These two personnel spent the early spring learning the basics of digital video. The first live broadcast event from the library's equipment was of the Eccles Library InfoFair 2000 keynote speaker. InfoFair is an event held at the library each year, bringing in notable speakers on current topics, usually relating to innovative use of technology in the health sciences. That year, the theme was "Video Visions: Integrating Multimedia in the Curriculum."[30] Other than the inability to turn off the digital camera time stamp display, leaving that unsightly mess on the screen throughout the broadcast, it was a relative success. Later, investigation of the camera's manual informed the staff that the camera's remote control allows the hiding of the time stamp. The lecture was broadcast live and archived for later viewing. The lecture relied heavily on a large screen projected from the speaker's computer. The projected presentation was captured by shooting the large screen display with the digital camera. The quality of this indirect capture was poor. It was also difficult to control the quality of the sound when taking the feed directly from the microphone.

To better capture sound and computer images used by a presenter, the library purchased an audio switcher and a computer-to-video scan converter. With these additions, the video image could be switched between the digital video camera and the computer, capturing the speaker with the camera and the image directly from the presenter's computer. This provided much greater clarity for any image coming from the computer, although the 320×240 display limits clarity when displaying a Web page or detailed PowerPoint slide. The sound mixer allowed more control over the sound coming in and facilitated making adjustments as necessary during an event.

Moving the entire server, monitor, and all the accompanying equipment was ungainly. The entire collection of hardware had been placed on an existing metal library cart with small wheels. Most routes out of the building required either hoisting the cart full of expensive equipment up and down a short flight of stairs, or using a ramp that had ruts and bumps that sent the monitor reeling. After a few near crashes, a new solution was designed. A powerful laptop was used to capture the video and send it back to the server, stored permanently at the library. This arrangement required that RealProducer be installed on the mobile laptop, sending the video over the network to the RealServer on the stationary server. A closeable case with an internal rack, like those used by traveling rock bands, was purchased to allow all the equipment to be bolted in, ready to use, and stable enough to be shipped if needed. All the necessary equipment was now moved in one low, wheeled shipping case. This greatly enhanced the system's mobility and decreased set up time and complexity.

The weekly Medical Informatics seminar and a graduate nursing statistics class were the first weekly broadcast events. A set of issues were encountered while doing the mobile broadcasts. Some rooms scheduled for broadcasting had only one network port, creating a conflict between the video broadcast and the presenter's need for Internet access. In other cases, the network port was at the front of the auditorium and network cable had to be strung the entire length of the room to connect the broadcast equipment located in the back. It was discovered that the network connections around the Health Sciences Center varied dramatically in bandwidth throughput. Some rooms would not retain a broadcast for more than a few minutes without dropping the connection; others were more stable. While broadcasting the second annual InfoFair in 2001, the venue experienced a network drop during the final minutes of the keynote lecture. Without hesitation, the broadcast was restarted, only to discover that the archive was overwritten through this action. The entire program archive was lost.

To prevent another unfortunate loss, the library incorporated yet another piece of equipment into the sleek mobile unit. All video and audio feeds were looped through a digital tape deck, capturing the entire presentation on tape, as well as attempting to archive live. In this way, if anything happened to the archive, it could be re-captured from tape. Using RealProducer, this could be done in real time, so a one-hour lecture could be re-captured to RealMedia format in one hour. The file would also have to be moved to the server and links prepared for viewers to reach the video. This provided a good safeguard to prevent total loss of the archive.

Today, the tape system has been replaced with a FireWire hard drive. The stream can be encoded as it is broadcast, creating the archive file for uploading immediately after the event. This provides a quick turnaround for availability of on-demand viewing. Additionally, the program can be recorded in raw video, allowing for post-processing into any format required by the client.

Following the disaster of September 11, 2001, network security began to take on a new focus. With the 2002 Olympics coming to Salt Lake City, many high security measures were implemented in an effort to prevent disruptive events during this high profile event. This resulted in many unexpected impacts on video broadcasting. It became a common occurrence to set up the broadcast unit in a classroom, only to find all broadcasting and video ports were blocked from network traffic. Many meetings with the Health Sciences Center IT department led to designation of specific rooms for broadcasting, with high bandwidth video VLANs set aside for broadcasting from those rooms. This created a significant limitation on where the mobile service could be deployed. This problem was solved when a new educational facility was built on the Health Sciences campus.

In the fall of 2005, a new state of the art Health Sciences Education Building was opened on the University of Utah campus adjacent to the library building. The Eccles Health Sciences Library manages the classroom technology for the building. This includes 31 classrooms of various sizes, as well as lab and clinical skills areas. The classrooms in this new building were planned to accommodate digital video. Each classroom has ports for capturing the computer displays and audio at the back of the room. The mobile unit can be quickly rolled into the classroom, plugged in and ready to go in a matter of minutes. This, combined with the growth in distance education and the general acceptance of video as a means of distributing and archiving course content, has led to a dramatic increase in use of the library's video services. The Medical Informatics seminars continue to be broadcast.

During the 2005-06 academic year, 304 video events were produced at the health sciences center, primarily taking place in the new education building. These events included standard course lecture broadcast and archiving, special event broadcasts, small group work, patient interviews, and special events. There were 119 events for the School of Medicine, 148 for the College of Nursing, and 37 for the College of Pharmacy. The trend continues, as 249 events have been scheduled for the fall 2006 semester alone, covering August through December.

On-Demand, Archival Digital Video Projects at Eccles Library

In addition to the broadcasting service, the library provided conversion and original video production services. In the summer of 2000, a collection of eye movement disorders was converted from VHS tape for Kathleen B. Digre, MD, a faculty member in the John A. Moran Eye Center's Neuro-Ophthalmology unit at the University of Utah. These highly specialized video clips were ideally suited to digital format. The information was uniquely visual, the clips were relatively short, and they had good narrative audio descriptions. Many of the cases were extremely rare examples of disorders that are infrequently seen in clinics, so made excellent teaching examples for medical students, residents, and fellows. The popularity of this collection led to the National Library of Medicine (NLM) grant-funded Neuro-Ophthalmology Virtual Education Library, or NOVEL,[31] project, which now contains more than 200 specialized medical videos showing neuro-ophthalmic disorders.

NOVEL has provided the Eccles Library with experience in dealing with video as information resources, from production to access. Each video is produced in five formats to provide maximum ease of access for users. Two streaming formats are intended to provide users with preview capabilities. Larger, higher quality formats are produced for download. The video clips in NOVEL are all entered into the digital asset management system used by the University of Utah, CONTENTdm. Each of these new collections must be described and indexed so that library users can find them. Assigning metadata has provided some interesting challenges, depending on the complexity of the video. Where in some cases a brief description is adequate, in other cases the metadata is serving as a case report. Each video is described and can be searched within the NOVEL collections, and through the larger digital library collection of the University. In addition, the NOVEL collection has a record in the online catalog and in the University of Utah's Institutional Repository.

Additional original production and conversion projects included creating a patient education tutorial,[32] taping neurologic examinations, digitizing psychiatric interviews, and converting a series of history of medicine at the University of Utah tapes. Each conversion project requires appropriate input devices. The library's technical staff was surprised at the volume of materials still stored on 3/4" tapes. One challenge has been to preserve the necessary input devices as they have become obsolete. Most of these video files are hosted on the library's video server and are accessible to the world. As the library builds its Institutional Repository,[33] faculty video collections will be added as they are identified.

USE IN THE NATIONAL NETWORK OF LIBRARIES OF MEDICINE (NN/LM) MIDCONTINENTAL REGION (MCR)

The MidContinental Region (MCR) of the National Network of Libraries of Medicine (NN/LM) sought to offer its members live and on-demand video streaming events and classes so that member librarians could view the events regardless of location and time constraints. The MCR planned to ship the Eccles Library mobile video broadcasting unit described above to its resource libraries so that trained staff at the resource libraries could broadcast events to the region. Resource libraries did not need to have access to a streaming server; the video was encoded on the fly during the event at the resource library and sent over the Internet to the Eccles Library Helix streaming video server.

From 2003-2005, one of the authors (SD) conducted training sessions at three resource libraries in advance of live events. Initially the training was conducted using the large mobile video broadcasting unit; this proved too unwieldy and difficult to ship without incurring damage to the unit. Later training sessions utilized the "mini" mobile unit, which was easier to assemble and less costly to ship.

Over the course of two years, four training sessions and subsequent broadcast events were offered to the region. Several of the live broadcasts failed due to technical reasons; however, four events were recorded and are available on the MCR Web site for on-demand viewing.[34] The topics covered by the events were of interest to health professionals (e.g.,

"Vitamins, Herbs and Alternative Supplements") or to librarians (e.g., Wyoming Symposium Hospital Libraries Panel).

After evaluating the results of the training sessions and member participation in the broadcast events, the program was suspended in mid-2005. Barriers to the program's success included:

- Although the mobile units are easy to assemble for an audiovisual technician who is accustomed to the equipment and configures it on a regular basis, it was difficult for library staff to assemble when they had not worked with the equipment for several months. Set-up, testing, and disassembly proved time-consuming even for the trained librarians.
- Without day-to-day experience working with the equipment and software, troubleshooting problems on the fly during a live broadcast was difficult and stressful.
- A number of factors beyond the control of the resource library could lead to a failed live broadcast. For instance, resource libraries needed to have a high bandwidth Internet connection available for the encoded file to be sent to the Eccles Library streaming server; but interruptions or unexpected slowness in local Internet service during an event might lead to a failed broadcast. One failure occurred when the Eccles Library server was overloaded due to a broadcast at the University of Utah happening at the same time as the resource library broadcast.
- Resource libraries did not always see value in investing the time and staff needed to offer video streaming services.
- Member libraries, particularly hospital librarians, often could not access the live broadcasts or the on-demand video due to bandwidth constraints, strict firewall configurations, or institutional rules preventing them from installing the RealMedia software.
- Members who were able to connect were often frustrated when a broadcast failed due to Internet or server problems. After a few failed broadcasts, they did not see the service as being reliable and were reluctant to tune in to the next event.

Despite these results, the MCR continues to believe that online video services are a useful method to provide "anytime, anywhere" distance education opportunities to member libraries. Video technology on the Internet is rapidly becoming ubiquitous, and at the same time video equipment and production software is becoming smaller, cheaper, and easier to use. In the future, the video services offered by the MCR may reflect these changes and take new forms, such as video podcasting or Flash videos served from online servers such as Google Video or YouTube.

CONCLUSION

Streaming and on-demand progressive download media are becoming ubiquitous on the Web. Video is no longer seen as something "extra" or unique on a Web site but rather as an integral part of the Web site content.[35]

Users are accessing video "on the go" with portable video devices such as the Apple Video iPod and even cell phones. In addition to consuming video content, users are also now contributing their own video content to Web sites such as YouTube and Google video. As of July 2006, 100 million video clips were viewed daily on YouTube, with 65,000 new videos uploaded every 24 hours.[36]

As the younger generation moves into academic and hospital library settings, they will expect access to streaming and on-demand video content. Health sciences librarians can become technology innovators within their institutions by offering streaming media services in support of research, patient care, and education.

REFERENCES

1. Crow, S., and Ondrusek, A. "Video as a Format in Health Information." *Medical Reference Services Quarterly* 21(Fall 2002): 21-34.

2. Brown, L. "Streaming Video: The Wave of the Video Future!" *Library Media Connection* 23(November/December 2004): 54-5.

3. Ross, J. "Streaming Video: Why to Do It, How to Do It, and Where to Get It." *MultiMedia & Internet@Schools* 12(September/October 2005): 9-11.

4. Valenza, J. "Animate Learning with Digital Video." *School Library Journal* 52(September 2006): 24.

5. Hickok, J. "Web Library Tours: Using Streaming Video And Interactive Quizzes." *Reference Services Review* 30(2002): 99-111.

6. Lee, S., and Burrell, C. "Introduction to Streaming Video for Novices." *Library Hi Tech News* 21(2004): 20-4.

7. Crowther, Karmen N. T., and Wallace, Alan H. "Creating and Delivering Video Streamed Orientation and Instruction on the Internet." 20th Annual Conference on Distance Teaching and Learning, 2005.

8. Cox, C., and Pratt, S. "The Case of the Missing Students, and How We Reached Them with Streaming Media." *Computers in Libraries* 22(March 2002): 40-5.

9. Maness, J.M. "An Evaluation of Library Instruction Delivered to Engineering Students Using Streaming Video." *Issues in Science and Technology Librarianship* (Summer 2006). Available: <http://www.istl.org/06-summer/refereed.html>. Accessed: November 20, 2006.

10. Tempelman-Kluit, N., and Ehrenberg, E. "Library Instruction and Online Tutorials: Developing Best Practices for Streaming Desktop Video Capture." *Feliciter* 49(2003): 89-90.

11. Yi Xiao, D.; Pietraszewski, B.; and Goodwin, S.P. "Full Stream Ahead: Database Instruction Through Online Videos." *Library Hi Tech* 22(2004): 366-74.

12. Barillari, J. "Satellite and Streaming Video: A Producer's View." *American Libraries* 37(June/July 2006): 48-9.

13. MLA Education. Available: <http://www.mlanet.org/education/>. Accessed: November 20, 2006.

14. Abram, S. "Islands in the Stream." *Information Outlook* 10(July 2006): 38-9.

15. RealNetworks Media Servers. Available: <http://www.realnetworks.com/products/media_delivery.html>. Accessed: November 20, 2006.

16. Windows Media Streaming Server. Available: <http://www.microsoft.com/windows/windowsmedia/howto/articles/webserver.aspx>. Accessed: November 20, 2006.

17. Apple QuickTime Streaming Server. Available: <http://www.apple.com/quicktime/streamingserver/>. Accessed: November 20, 2006.

18. Developer Connection. Open Source Darwin Streaming Server. Available: <http://developer.apple.com/opensource/server/streaming/index.html/>. Accessed: November 20, 2006.

19. Adobe Flash Media Server. Available: <http://www.adobe.com/products/flashmediaserver//>. Accessed: November 20, 2006.

20. Horizon Wimba. Available: <http://www.horizonwimba.com/>. Accessed: November 20, 2006.

21. RealMedia Player. Available: <http://www.real.com>. Accessed: November 20, 2006.

22. Microsoft Windows Media Player. Available: <http://www.microsoft.com/windows/windowsmedia/default.mspx>. Accessed: November 20, 2006.

23. Apple QuickTime Player. Available: <http://www.apple.com/quicktime/download/win.html>. Accessed: November 20, 2006.

24. Adobe Flash Player. Available: <http://www.adobe.com/products/flashplayer/>. Accessed: November 20, 2006.

25. Sorenson Services USA Video Bandwidth Estimator. Available: <http://sorenson-usa.com/vbe/index.html>. Accessed: November 20, 2006.

26. Codec Guide for the MIT Computer Graphics Group. (October 23, 2003). Available: <http://people. csail.mit.edu/tbuehler/video/codecs/index.html>. Accessed: November 20, 2006.

27. Virginia Tech Faculty Development Workshop. (Fall 2002). Available: <http://www.fdi.vt.edu/fall/2002/s_content/streaming/technical.html>. Accessed: November 20, 2006.

28. Nielsen, Jakob. "Talking Head Video is Boring." *Alertbox* (December 5, 2005). Available: <http://www.useit.com/alertbox/video.html>. Accessed: November 20, 2006.

29. Adams, J. "The Part Played by Instructional Media in Distance Education." *Simile* 6(May 2006): 1.

30. "Video Visions: Integrating Multimedia in the Curriculum." *InfoFair* (2000). Available: <http://library.med.utah.edu/or/infofair/infofair.php>. Accessed: November 20, 2006.

31. Neuro-Ophthalmology Virtual Education Library: NOVEL. Available: <http://library.med.utah.edu/NOVEL/>. Accessed: November 20, 2006.

32. Patient Education Workshop. Available: <http://library.med.utah.edu/Patient_Ed/>. Accessed: November 20, 2006.

33. University of Utah Institutional Repository. Available: <http://ir.utah.edu>. Accessed: November 20, 2006.

34. National Network of Library of Medicine Mid-Continental Region Web Site. Available: <http://nnlm.gov/mcr/>. Accessed: November 20, 2006.

35. Green, T. "The Rise of Flash Video, Part 1." *Digital Web Magazine* (October 2006). Available: <http://www.digital-web.com/articles/the_rise_of_flash_video_part_1/>. Accessed: November 20, 2006.

36. "YouTube Serves Up 100 Million Videos a Day Online." *USA Today, Gannett Co. Inc.* (July 2006). Available: <http://www.usatoday.com/tech/news/2006-07-16-youtube-views_x.htm>. Accessed: November 20, 2006.

doi:10.1300/J115v26S01_06

Social Networking

Melissa L. Rethlefsen

SUMMARY. The major social networking tools like MySpace and Facebook give people an online identity–and an online space to call their own. Other social networking tools are more nuanced than sharing whole personalities like on MySpace. Tools like LibraryThing, Flickr, and del.icio.us that focus on connecting people through certain media and interests offer specialized value to users. This paper describes major social networking, social media sharing, and social bookmarking tools; what they are used for; and how libraries and librarians are using them. Tagging, a concept critical to social bookmarking and social media sharing, and folksonomy are discussed in relation to these tools. doi:10.1300/ J115v26S01_07 *[Article copies available for a fee from The Haworth Document Delivery Service: 1-800-HAWORTH. E-mail address: <docdelivery@ haworthpress.com> Website: <http://www.HaworthPress.com> © 2007 by The Haworth Press, Inc. All rights reserved.]*

KEYWORDS. Social networking, social bookmarking, social software, tagging, folksonomy, MySpace, Facebook, Vox, Flickr, LibraryThing, YouTube, del.icio.us

---

Melissa L. Rethlefsen, MLS (mlrethlefsen@gmail.com) is an education technology librarian, Mayo Clinic College of Medicine, 200 First Street SW, Rochester, MN 55905.

[Haworth co-indexing entry note]: "Social Networking." Rethlefsen, Melissa L. Co-published simultaneously in *Medical Reference Services Quarterly* (The Haworth Information Press, an imprint of The Haworth Press, Inc.) Vol. 26, Supp. #1, 2007, pp. 117-141; and: *Medical Librarian 2.0: Use of Web 2.0 Technologies in Reference Services* (ed: M. Sandra Wood) The Haworth Information Press, an imprint of The Haworth Press, Inc., 2007, pp. 117-141. Single or multiple copies of this article are available for a fee from The Haworth Document Delivery Service [1-800-HAWORTH, 9:00 a.m. - 5:00 p.m. (EST). E-mail address: docdelivery@haworthpress.com].

INTRODUCTION

From the chaff of fallen dotcoms, Geocities pages, and the static Web has arisen a new day of consumer empowerment on the Internet. Though connecting and sharing have always been a major part of the Web, all the way from the days of Usenet and multiplayer BBS games, users rather than products have now taken a place of utmost importance in the Web's shape. Called Web 2.0, this new era of flexible platforms, consumer content creation, and user development has shaken up what the Web means. Along with new ways of presenting and releasing content via AJAX, open APIs, and lightweight programming backends, Web content has morphed from merely publications to providing possibilities for participation and rich user experience. Web 2.0 services depend inherently upon the user to add value by creating content and acting as developers, relying on the premise that users collectively can be trusted to produce great things. As Tim O'Reilly says in his seminal article, "What is Web 2.0," "Hyperlinking is the foundation of the web. As users add new content, and new sites, it is bound in to the structure of the web by other users discovering the content and linking to it. Much as synapses form in the brain, with associations becoming stronger through repetition or intensity, the web of connections grows organically as an output of the collective activity of all web users."[1]

Because of its reliance on users to provide content and value, Web 2.0 services are largely social software, which can be construed as any software tool or Web application that facilitates communication, sharing, collaboration, or the creation of community online. In this vein, older tools like Usenet, bulletin boards, and Internet Relay Chat are social software; in fact, the term social software dates to 1987, though it entered common usage in 2002.[2] With the advent of Web 2.0 tools and ideology, however, new services and tools have come to epitomize social software: wikis, blogs, instant messaging, social networking tools, social bookmarking, and more. Key to all of these applications is the user.

ORIGINS AND HISTORY
OF SOCIAL NETWORKING APPLICATIONS

Like social software, social networking has a longer history than its recent buzzword status would imply. From Classmates.com to dating Web sites like Match.com to LiveJournal, many Web sites dating from the mid-1990s capitalized on creating online communities and finding people with like interests. Sites explicitly dedicated to social networking like Six Degrees and SocialNet died without fanfare in the late 1990s.[3] But when Friendster was introduced in 2002 and rocketed to popularity in 2003, social networking became a major player on the Web. Today, pure social networking sites like MySpace and Facebook, along with specialized social networking services like YouTube, Flickr, Digg, and del.icio.us rank amongst the United States' and the world's favorite places to go on the Web.[4,5] MySpace itself ranks as the third most popular destination for American Web surfers–coming in only after Google and Yahoo!–and sixth worldwide, garnering millions of visitors daily. Estimates range between 37.8 and 56.8 million unique visitors traversing MySpace's pages per day.[6,7]

Social networking application developers, beginning with Six Degrees, built upon offline social networking concepts when designing their products. Whether using the theory of six degrees of separation or the belief that the average person has 150 friends, the social networking sites planned to create value in their products by helping people to articulate and exploit those degrees of separation online, whether for dating, finding jobs, or meeting people. Indeed, Friendster, the pioneer of successful online social networking, states in its recently awarded patent, "What is needed is a system that allows individuals to replicate the process of developing personal relationships through social networks, using a computer system and database. The system should calculate and display social networks in a way that lets people better manage and exploit their own social networks."[8]

Popular social networking tools today focus less on degrees of separation and more on giving people ways to share with each other. The major social networking tools like MySpace and Facebook give people an online identity–and an online space to call their own. Other social networking tools are more nuanced than sharing whole personalities like on MySpace. Tools like LibraryThing, Flickr, and del.icio.us that focus on connecting people through certain media and interests offer specialized value to users, whether in finding great images or books, or keeping up to date with what's happening in the news. These sites are all about community participation.

SOCIAL NETWORKING

"It is the 21st century, and we are all each other's Hummel figurines."
–Lore Sjöberg[9]

Social networking sites generally have two primary components: a user profile and a network of friends. A user profile consists at the very least of a name or username, but more often is a detailed list of a user's personal information and preferences, plus photographs, music, videos, animated graphics, and anything else an individual adds to spice up his or her page. The friends network, however, is the real key to social networking sites–the crux of what differentiates them from blogs, online journals, personal Web sites, and other means of personal communication on the Web. The number and quality of one's friends on MySpace, Facebook, or a similar site is essentially a form of social currency, in addition to providing an easy means to keep up to date with what one's friends are doing and saying.[10] Finding friends is usually just as simple as searching or browsing the Web site, requesting to be someone's friend, and having that request accepted or turned down.

"Friending" someone online is not exactly the same as actually being a person's friend in reality–social networking friends may be personal friends, acquaintances, co-workers, classmates, celebrities, or even commodities. Musicians in particular have made use of sites like MySpace to promote themselves, increasing their reach into pop culture by accepting as many friends as possible. MySpace has become such a massive marketing tool for musicians that there are even online guides teaching musicians how to make the most of MySpace.[11] One comedian, Dane Cook, famously catapulted his previously lackluster career into stardom using MySpace–he gathered over 1 million friends in his network and used it to self-promote all of his performances and products.[12]

MySpace

"If the internet had no myspace, i would not even bother"[13]

As noted above, MySpace is currently and overwhelmingly the most popular social networking site in the world. What makes MySpace so special? Its sheer size and market share are now the number one reason it is so popular. Teens and college students, for example, often state that they "have" to be on MySpace in order to keep up with their friends. But, why did people start gravitating to MySpace in the first place? MySpace, unlike Friendster, which suffered from stagnation, had a lot that users could do. As an article in *Newsweek* put it, "[MySpace] concentrated on building a site that easily allowed users to create their own little online treehouses, adding photos, videos, music and blogs."[12] A typical MySpace page includes all of these components, plus an extensive comment wall where friends can communicate. "It's just an amazing site that really makes the world feel a lot smaller," said one dedicated user.[13]

MySpace is often criticized by those with even a modicum of taste for its frantic and chaotic pages; a satirical personal testimonial in *Wired News* gleefully announced, "Looking at randomly selected MySpaces, I discover that one of the most important things to do with your page is embed random crap from other places on the web. Ha! Easy!"[9] In a more positive review, *Business Week* recently called MySpace "unfettered design chaos," noting that "user pages on MySpace can look truly hideous (and many, many of them do)," but simultaneously recognizing that the amateurish look of MySpace is the key to its success. It allows those with no professional design skill and no Web experience to customize their own space without feeling intimidated.[14]

MySpace, however, faces intense criticism of another kind; there is deep concern that MySpace and other social networking tools expose children and teenagers' personal information and make them vulnerable to predators. In response to this concern, Rep. Michael Fitzpatrick [R-PA] drafted a bill called "Deleting Online Predators Act of 2006," or DOPA.[15] This bill, which the House of Representatives passed 410 to 15 on July 26, 2006 despite the protestations of the American Library Association and many others, requires schools and libraries to block minor access to social networking Web sites, including MySpace, to receive funding.[16] As of November 15, 2006, this bill had not yet been heard in the Senate committee to which it was referred.

DOPA caused great outcry in the library and educational communities because of its overly broad language and restrictions. Children and Young Adult librarians are particularly vociferous in their opposition to DOPA. The YALSA (Young Adult Library Services Association) Blog was one of those voices, demonstrating 30 positive uses of social networking in an October 2006 series.[17] These uses spanned across the social networking board to include tools like Digg, del.icio.us, YouTube, Second Life, and others, but also specifically addressed the positive aspects of MySpace for teens and libraries. Some of their MySpace examples included networking with authors, boosting teen participation in the library, and using MySpace bulletins to market events.

In fact, most libraries currently using MySpace are using it to market library events and library services. For example, one of the longest running library MySpace sites, the Hennepin County Library, has blogged about an upcoming DDR (Dance Dance Revolution) night, Teen Read Month, and blogging classes. The Brooklyn College Library advertises upcoming library classes, as does the Perry-Castaneda Library (University of Texas at Austin). Many library MySpace sites link to library catalogs (Hennepin County, the UIUC Undergraduate Library, and the

Denver Public Library have search boxes built into their sites), library research guides, and library virtual or chat reference services. Several libraries focus on friending authors their patrons would enjoy; for instance, the Hennepin County Library and the Denver Public Library's MySpace sites friend young adult authors. One clever piece of marketing from the NJIT Library was to get students and alumni to answer one of eight questions about the library correctly in order to be listed in one of the top eight friends slots.[18]

But MySpace can be about more than marketing. It is also a way to connect with library patrons in a way not possible before. Beth Evans of the Brooklyn College Library writes,

> Investing some time in this new social network can really pay dividends. In traditional or even some newer reference environments, such as at the physical reference desk or in chat sessions, we tend to learn little about our patrons. . . . Reading student profiles [in MySpace] allows us to be a little playful with students and in some cases teach them about the library without their even asking for such information. For example, we suggested one student track down a certain call number after offering a small bit of virtual instruction in using the online catalog. The student followed the suggestion and was delighted to discover that the call number led him to his favorite book.[19]

Though some might wonder if the MySpace bubble is about to burst, especially in light of recent news articles like the *Washington Post*'s "In Teens World, MySpace Is So Last Year"[20] and the *Wall Street Journal*'s "MySpace ByeSpace"[21] sounding MySpace's death knell, it is clear MySpace is here to stay, at least for now. Indeed, recent statistics show that MySpace has already accrued so much mainstream popularity that adults over 35 are visiting the site in large numbers, though not necessarily with the time and energy commitment its key user groups currently spend.[22] And the demise of MySpace and social networking sites seems to have been greatly exaggerated by journalists; LeeAnn Prescott of Hitwise, a Web traffic monitoring company, rebutted their claims, stating that though "it has been reported that there was a decline in visits to sites like MySpace and Facebook in September [2006]," it "is a typical seasonal occurrence as school-aged users shift their attention from socializing online to academic pursuits."[23]

In the recent Medical Library Association Webcast, "Moving at the Speed of Byte," one panelist mentioned that MySpace is not as appropriate for medical libraries as for public libraries because it is largely a purview of teenagers.[24] Since teenagers are quick to become college students, medical students, residents, and doctors, however, academic medical libraries and other medical libraries should be familiar with MySpace and how it will impact libraries in the future.

Facebook

"Facebook is like crack. We've all known this for approximately two years and change now."–Dr. Date to Logged Off, a student whose girlfriend spends all her time on Facebook[25]

Facebook is the second most popular social networking Web site in the United States.[4] Originally designed for college students at a limited number of schools, Facebook slowly opened up its services to high schools, corporations, and finally, on September 26, 2006, Facebook opened its site to the world.[26] Facebook is a social networking site with an interesting twist. Unlike MySpace, which is a vast open network, Facebook creates siloed networks for regions, schools, or corporations. Having siloed networks means that information is marginally more private; for instance, a student at the University of Minnesota would not be able to see a University of Michigan student's Facebook unless a friend relationship existed. Without a Facebook account, nothing is visible.

Facebook is massively popular with college students; studies have shown that 85% to 94.4% of students at supported institutions have Facebook accounts.[27-30] Not only do students have accounts, but they really use them; 60% of those students log on daily.[30] Anecdotal evidence and personal experience show that students are logging in while in class, while more concrete studies have shown that some students are logging in for hours each day or checking their accounts and their friends' pages hourly.[29,31]

Facebook hit a particular niche that finds its service indispensable. Fred Stutzman, a PhD student researching Facebook, argues,

> The Facebook is truly a killer app for incoming freshmen–as they prepare to start a new life in a new place, surrounded by a new social network, the Facebook presents a highly interactive way to explore this new space. For those of us who sent snail-mail letters to our freshman year roommates, Facebook is everything we could have dreamed of and then some–not only can students know everything about their new roommates, but they can learn everything

about their suite, their floor, and their dorm. This is information students need to know, and it helps them get situated in their new social networks.[28]

Stutzman believes that Facebook's success is due to "situational relevance," the idea that Facebook fills a particular need for a particular group in a particular situation. He persuasively notes, "For the college student, their world is largely the campus; the Facebook provides a constant companion as they navigate the college experience."[32] Undergraduates are not the only ones using Facebook, however; a quick check for Mayo Medical School students showed 29 of 43 first-year and 23 of 42 second-year students with active Facebook accounts.

In addition to the gated and siloed networks, Facebook operates differently than other social networking tools. One of its main selling points for college students and other users alike is photo sharing. Facebook allows users to post an unlimited number of photos to the site, the only limit being that there can only be 60 photos per album. This is a big difference from other social networking sites like MySpace, which make users upload content elsewhere (e.g., Flickr or Photobucket) where limits to number of uploads or cost make it harder to share. All Facebook photos can be tagged with people's names as well, meaning that a person can instantly see all pictures of herself that any friends have posted and tagged. Facebook also incorporates a limited type of social bookmarking called My Shares (basically, a way to send links to friends), the ability to import and syndicate an RSS feed of choice, an events calendar, and hundreds of groups focusing on politics to classes to personal interests to just plain amusement. For example, the group "Wikipedia is helping me get through med school!" has over 1,200 members.

Facebook's popularity continues to grow—their traffic was up 16% in October 2006, despite the intense criticism it drew from some of its biggest fans in September 2006.[23] On September 4, 2006, Facebook introduced "news feeds," an updating stream of information about a user's friends' every action, from a change in relationship status to posting a comment on someone's "wall."[33] Instead of reacting to this change with pleasure, as Facebook had anticipated, a wellspring of resentment and anger surged up in resistance to what Facebook aficionados saw as an affront to their privacy.[34] Over 700,000 people—almost one-tenth of Facebook's members—signed up for the "Students Against Facebook News Feeds" group, and the Facebook creators were forced to scramble to put together some privacy options. With the new privacy options in place, Facebook appears to have bounced back and regained its place as second only to iPods and tied with beer in American college popular culture.[35]

Academic libraries and librarians were quick to start using Facebook in many of the same ways libraries use MySpace: marketing the library and library services, promoting events, and connecting with users. One librarian, Brian Mathews at the Georgia Institute of Technology Library, used Facebook to send a message to 1,500 students, receiving in return 48 Facebook messages back with questions about the library, instant messages asking for help finding journal articles, and several "friend" requests.[36] The Georgia Institute of Technology Library also used Facebook to market their 2006 freshman orientation, CeLIBration @ the GT Library.[37] To market this event, the library created Facebook events and sent out focused invitations. For example, the library invited single students interested in dating to the speed dating event, students interested in playing tag or in ninjas to the ninja tag event, and students interested in retro gaming to do some old school gaming. In addition, the library purchased advertising space on Facebook for the three days prior to the event.[38] Commenting on the success of the Facebook event for retro gamers, Mathews noted, "FaceBook[sic] should give me an endorsement deal. Once more we were able to target students with interest in gaming. Of all the activities we promoted, this one received the more[sic] buzz. Student posting[sic] several comments to each other and there was tremendous excitement before they arrived."[39] Another library, the Crossett Library at Bennington College, used their Facebook account for collection development purposes, finding students' favorite books and movies, purchasing them for the library when possible, and alerting the student.[40]

In recent months, a great deal of ire has sprung up towards Facebook from librarians, however, because Facebook began systematically deleting all profiles for "non-human entities."[41] As recorded by Beth Kraemer at the University of Kentucky, in September 2006, there were 76 libraries using Facebook; by October 25, 2006, there were only three.[42] Whether or not this proves to be a large mistake for Facebook remains unknown, but since killing the "fakesters"–fake accounts, groups, institutions, etc.–led to the demise of Friendster, Facebook is treading on shaky ground. In response to the outcry, Stutzman articulated the errors of Facebook's ways:

> Do we really need to discuss how much damage actions like these cause to a social network? Does Facebook somehow think that it is not susceptible to the mistakes made by other social networks? Is it

possible Facebook thinks it is above failure? Lets[sic] make this very clear: the murder of the fakesters was the single biggest component leading to the downfall of Friendster. I can't believe they are doing it at Facebook. . .

When the fakester is killed, social capital and connectedness are lost in the network. Librarians who have worked hard to publicize their libraries[sic] work, and the users who depend on them are suddenly disconnected. For many of them, they will never reconnect. That bond in the network is lost, and the network becomes substantially less valuable.

What Friendster didn't realize, and Facebook seems like it doesn't realize, is that fakesters are real. Your social networks are made up of people and objects–both serve important roles connecting us.[43]

Though Facebook has not yet budged on the library issue, Mathews is working with Chief Revenue Officer Mike Murphy about the value libraries offer the Facebook networks. Should institutional profiles remain banned, there are still many ways for librarians to participate and connect with patrons in Facebook. Mathews suggests that subject librarians set up personal accounts and use those to connect with students.[44] Libraries can also set up a library group or groups, perhaps focusing on particular classes, assignments, or library services. Paid advertising is another option.

Overall, Facebook appears to be very well positioned to keep students coming for years to come. Whether it can capitalize as effectively on its new audiences remains to be seen, but it is so pervasive on campuses that EDUCAUSE dedicated one of its *7 Things* series papers just to Facebook, stating that, "As users become more sophisticated and a broader population is represented online, students will start to use social networking sites to make professional connections with people through topics of deep intellectual interest to them."[45] Libraries should be there to help.

Vox

"No *one updates their LJ anymore. Vox is for, you know,* grown-ups." –H2[46]

Vox is a newer social networking site created by Six Apart, the same company that gave the world LiveJournal and Moveable Type. Vox is built on the premise that soon people will get sick of the lack of privacy options offered by MySpace and other social networking tools, but will still want and need to use social networking spaces to connect with friends, family, and others. What Vox promises to do is provide robust privacy options like its predecessor, LiveJournal, but with a Web 2.0 upgrade to the look, feel, and operation of the site. Vox was released to the general populace on October 25, 2006, but had 85,000 invitation-only Voxers before that release.[47]

In its brief life, Vox has already generated a lot of enthusiasm, including veritably glowing reviews on *Boing Boing, Wired News, O'Reilly Radar,* and *Techcrunch.* In large part, this is due to the privacy options Vox offers, though there is much more to Vox. For instance, Vox interacts with Amazon, providing a way to track the books and music a Vox user owns. Vox also provides apparently unlimited video, audio, and photo uploading, storage, and management. It operates smoothly with a number of online services many people already depend on: Amazon, Flickr, and YouTube, to name a few. Vox faces some stiff competition from another privacy-focused social networking site, Multiply, but with momentum from an already successful company, it could go far.

More Social Networking Sites. Hi5, Cyworld, Tagworld, Bebo, Windows Live Spaces, Yahoo 360, imeem, and orkut are all social networking sites ranging from the up and coming to the well established. Many of these sites are very popular outside of the United States; for instance, Cyworld is dominated by Asia–traffic is primarily from Korea, Taiwan, and Japan. orkut, a site owned by Google, is especially popular, even potentially competing with MySpace, though two-thirds or more of its members are Brazilian.[48] As social networking tools fade in and out of vogue, any of these could prove major competition to MySpace.

Social Networking in Education

Social networking tools are gaining recognition in educational circles for their potential to engage students creatively and thoughtfully, as well as to establish a record of a student's progress through their coursework. As mentioned above, EDUCAUSE sees Facebook as one potential venue for such creativity, and in fact, some course instructors are communicating with their students via Facebook's private group options. Vox, due to its privacy restrictions, has also been mentioned as a potential tool for education, as has LiveJournal, for the same reasons.[49,50] Education's killer social networking application, however, may be Elgg.

Elgg is an open source social networking system designed specifically for educators and students to use as an e-portfolio, blogging, sharing, and collaboration tool.[51] Like LiveJournal and Vox, Elgg is fraught with granular privacy options; students can decide who can see each individual post, photos, files, and more. Having been designed with education in mind, Elgg plays nicely with other education applications like WebCT and Moodle. Elgg is already being used with great success by students and teachers in K-12 and higher education settings.[52-55] The Mayo Medical School, which currently uses LiveJournal, is considering switching to Elgg as an e-portfolio tool. Because it is open source, it can be launched anywhere for any group of students, educators, or even library staff. Elgg's creators also recently announced Elgg Spaces, a hosted application allowing users to create private Elgg domains without worrying about maintaining servers.

Enterprise Social Networking

Academic libraries are not the only libraries that should know about and be using social networking tools. Corporations, including hospitals, are very interested in social networking tools and applications. Why? In enterprise environments, sharing knowledge and finding experts is critical to the success of the organization. Social networking sites make it easy to find collaborators, along with providing users the tools to collaborate, like blogs, discussion boards, and more. Dissemination of knowledge is much easier in the kind of RSS-enabled push environments that social networking tools provide. Enterprise-scale social software applications currently range from the very specific (such as blogs, wikis, or social bookmarking) to the very broad, like Microsoft's SharePoint and its Knowledge Network add-on, which touts itself as a social networking and knowledge management tool.[56]

Everyone knows that a great deal of institutional knowledge lies in an institution's memory–specifically the minds of its employees. What SharePoint and other enterprise social networking tools hope to do is pull that knowledge from its employees' minds and put it where future workers and current colleagues can utilize it. SharePoint's Knowledge Network uses a unique way to establish its network; instead of relying on individuals to create and populate their own profiles, Knowledge Network "automatically builds profiles of employees and their areas of expertise" by spidering through e-mail and corporate Intranets.[56] Though this process sounds a bit Orwellian, individuals do get a chance to approve profiles before being posted, and all profile options, files, and other components have associated high-granularity privacy options for friends, boss, work unit, work group, and private postings.

IBM, a pioneer in enterprise social software creation, has been using an internal social networking tool, called Fringe, to leverage their organization's knowledge. Ten thousand users are already finding Fringe necessary to their daily work.[57] Fringe utilizes "people tagging," basically a tag cloud for an individual person that might represent skills, expertise, or current projects.[58] Fringe is now available as part of Lotus Connections, IBM's social software suite for enterprises. IBM's success points the way for Microsoft SharePoint and other competitors in enterprise social networking like Visible Path and Hoover's Connect.

Specialized Social Networking Tools

"Over time, I believe, people will get tired of the vast and generic theme of mainstream social networks–and move towards niche or vertical social networks that will serve their passions and interests."–Ebrahim Ezzy[59]

Many social networking experts see the future of social networking applications in smaller, tailored, or more private systems. Specialized social networking tools, which have the potential to target a particular niche audience or need, are already showing promise. One of the most successful tools is LinkedIn, a service designed for connecting business colleagues and networks. While nowhere near the traffic or reach of MySpace or Facebook, its traffic is on the rise, and the site has been profitable in recent months.[48,59] LinkedIn operates in much the same way as Friendster does, by building relationships between users by degrees (i.e., Sharon knows John (1st degree); John knows Sam (2nd degree); Sam knows Max (3rd degree)). Using the network, users can find business contacts, whether for finding jobs or just networking, by following the chains of contacts. LinkedIn also offers public and private groups; for instance, alumni organizations are using LinkedIn to provide a forum for alumni.

Much smaller scale specialty social networking applications are available. For the sciences, Nature Publishing Group has created the beta Nature Network Boston. Nature Network Boston offers free blogging tools for scientists, along with the ability to create networks and groups, and advertise events like upcoming research presentations. Currently, its user base is limited, but active. My Cancer Place is a social networking site for cancer patients, cancer survivors, and their families. Members can post photos, Web sites, blogs, and more in their personal profiles, as well as comment on others' profiles, join forums, take polls, and more. For patients, a social networking site like My Cancer Place is a way to feel less alone with their disease. Members take advantage of the camaraderie, building up friends networks with total strangers, posting encouraging comments on others' profiles, and engaging in discussion about many cancer topics.

SOCIAL MEDIA

Beyond social networking designed for specific communities are applications that are built around sharing specific types of media–already a large part of most major social networking sites. These specialty sites take media sharing much, much further. Flickr, the undisputed master of the social media genre, is the 38th most popular site in the world.[5] All social media sites are built around a few commonalities: personal collections, tagging and tag clouds, and ways to track other people's accounts, whether through friending, RSS, watch lists, or all of the above. These sites often don't get counted as social networking applications because of their focus on particular media, but most certainly are. As Stutzman says, "Social networks come in many forms–and many times those forms are much more nuanced than 'social network websites' where the explicit focus of the service is people."[60]

Flickr

"I've long been vocally skeptical of tagging's usefulness, but I have to admit what Flickr has done with tagging has impressed me."–Chris Sherman[61]

Flickr helps people share their photos with friends, family, customers, or the general public. Its design and technology has helped define what Web 2.0 technology means. Basic accounts on Flickr are free and offer the opportunity to display 200 photos; premium accounts, at $24.95 per year, offer unlimited, high-resolution storage. Like other social networking sites, Flickr utilizes user profiles and friends and family networks. By offering users both the right to limit who can see or use photos on an individual level and to set licensing rights for all images (e.g., Creative Commons), plus offering commenting and tagging functionality, Flickr has developed a large and loyal fan base. Tagging in particular helps users not only to organize their own photos, but to find other photos with the same tags. When people all upload photos from the same event, picking a standard tag like il2006 (Internet Librarian 2006) makes it easy to browse everyone's photos. Flickr's groups functionality likewise helps users "pool" their photos together, either privately or publicly.

Libraries and librarians have been some of Flickr's biggest supporters; the Libraries and Librarians group has over 1,000 members and a pool of over 6,000 photos. Michael Stephens, author of the *Tame the Web* blog, offers libraries 16 suggestions for using Flickr, including publicizing events, putting up photos of library staff, and presenting collections of historical images.[62] Others have suggested using Flickr as a digital collection repository.[63] Many of these suggestions have already been taken by libraries. From public libraries to medical libraries to librarians, Flickr is swarming with great library content. Some libraries are using Flickr to document library events, and some are using it to store screenshots and other images for use in blogs and publications. One medical library, the Health Sciences Library at Stony Brook University, posted images from training sessions, a lecture series, and of their library's patrons and architecture. A quick search for "ct scan" on Flickr produces dozens of results, mostly posted by patients. Searching can be limited to Creative Commons licensed photos, meaning Flickr is a great way to find images for presentations.

LibraryThing

"Oh. My. God. I have not been this excited about the Internet since I 'discovered' blogging. Have you seen that Library Thing?"–Danigirl[64]

Another amazing social media site is LibraryThing, a site where members catalog their book collections online. LibraryThing, like other social networking sites, offers users a personal profile, options to track other users' collections, and group and discussion functionality. Also a hit with librarians, LibraryThing is being used to catalog whole library collections, for collection development (finding book reviews and book recommendations), and even for putting updating lists and images of new books on library Web sites via RSS feeds.[65] LibraryThing, like Flickr, uses tagging to help users describe and organize their books. Each book has its own tag cloud which gives users detailed information about book content at a quick glance. LibraryThing is working on several projects with libraries; soon to be introduced is a service that allows libraries to build LibraryThing data, including tags, book reviews, and multiple edition information, and tagging directly into their OPACs.[66] With this move, LibraryThing will be poised to become a major player in the library world.

LibraryThing has several competitors in the social media cataloging game. Shelfari, aNobii, GuruLib, Socialogue, Listal, All Consuming, and imeem are a few of these, though none of them have LibraryThing's power or following. Shelfari and aNobii are book cataloging tools; GuruLib, Socialogue, Listal, and All Consuming add other types of media to books, including DVDs, movies, games, and music. imeem drops the books and adds photos, video sharing, and playlists; imeem also gives members blogs and the opportunity to syndicate blogs and RSS feeds from other sources, like MySpace profiles.

YouTube

"I am rich, rich I tells ya! Cuz as you heroes know, my show is all over the YouTube. You put my name into YouTube, you pull up over more than 2,600 videos. That's gotta be like a third of all their videos. That means I got $500 million coming to me!"–Stephen Colbert on hearing that Google bought YouTube for $1.65 billion

After YouTube was purchased by Google for $1.65 billion, YouTube became a household name. The service, which allows people to upload, stream, share, and rate videos, is incredibly popular. Recent cracking down on copyright means that finding last night's *Daily Show* may not be easy anymore, but anyone can still find plenty on YouTube, from short films like *Ryan vs. Dorkman* to the cell phone video footage of the UCLA student being tasered in the Powell Library. When *Time Magazine* awarded YouTube as its Invention of the Year, reporter Lev Grossman commented that "YouTube had tapped into something that appears on no business plan: the lonely, pressurized, pent-up video subconscious of America."[67]

YouTube has merit beyond entertainment. EDUCAUSE states,

> As a social-software application, YouTube is part of a trend among Net Generation students to replace passive learning with active participation, where everyone has a voice, anyone can contribute, and the value lies less in the content itself than in the networks of learners that form around content and support one another in learning goals.[68]

YouTube is already being used by libraries to fill some educational goals, such as posting video tours of the library, instructional videos, presentations, footage of library events, and more.

SOCIAL BOOKMARKING AND TAGGING

Social bookmarking sites offer another type of social networking to users. Instead of sharing photos, music, and videos, social bookmarkers share links, memes, articles, research, and other resources. Several types of social bookmarking services exist, from the basic bookmarking tools like del.icio.us, Ma.gnolia, and BlinkList, to tools like Furl that save copies of bookmarked Web pages, to academic social reference managers like Connotea, CiteULike, and Complore, to social annotation services like Diigo.[69,70] Social bookmarking services succeed based on one factor–they fill a personal need, the need to organize and store bookmarks better than can be done in a Web browser. They are so exciting because that need is not filled in a void. Social bookmarking tools allow users to explore serendipitous connections between their bookmarks and others', enabling discovery of new items and people with similar interests.

Social bookmarking has made its way into the library literature and blogosphere and libraries in force, in part due to its capability to share reference and reading lists, in part because it is a great way to store one's own personal bookmark collection–always being able to find a Web resource again is an excellent incentive for using social bookmarking tools–but in largest part due to the major backbone of social bookmarking, tagging. Tagging is also part of other social networking tools like Flickr, LibraryThing, and YouTube, though tagging's accomplice, folksonomy, is most often discussed with social bookmarking.

Tagging is simply the assigning of keywords to describe an item, whether a bookmark, photo, or piece of art. What makes tagging special is that anyone can do it with relatively little effort; each user assigns his own tags to any given item using keywords he thinks relevant either to himself or others for finding the item again. Because each individual user comes up with tags, tags vary widely across users. Many tags have personal or group meaning (toread, il2006, lis757, @home, for example), while other users have come up with complex tags using hierarchical folders, citing methods (using via: or cite:), and even Dublin Core.[71,72] Golder and Huberman defined seven major types of tags: (1) identifying what (or who) it is about (google, libraries, myspace); (2) identifying what it is (book, article, blogpost); (3) identifying who owns it (in:mashable, dc:creator=MillerPaul, slashdot); (4) refining categories (*, **, ***); (5) identifying qualities or characteristics (funny, crazy, kewl); (6) self reference (mycomments, me); and (7) task organizing (LS500_ Lecture10, finalpaper, forwork).[73] Even with the huge variance in tags and tagging styles, out of the masses of tags arises a folksonomy–a spontaneous and organic language of description and categorization.

Tagging, folksonomies, and their attendant technologies are already commonplace on the Web, spreading from the social bookmarking tools to being used to organize blogs, display large sets of data (for example, a tag cloud of a library catalog's subject headings), to Google's Co-op and Image Labeler projects, which let users tag Web sites and images, respectively. Enterprises have long seen the potential of tagging and social bookmarking for their institutions and Intranets. IBM, which also pioneered enterprise social networking with Fringe, created a social bookmarking network called Dogear.[74] Like other enterprise social networking applications, enterprise social bookmarking tools like Dogear, Cogenz, and ConnectBeam have the power to connect individuals with similar interests, but unlike basic social networking tools, also may develop as inroads into often poorly organized Intranets, either through search or by providing the basis for, or as input into, Intranet categorization and organization. Finding the terms employees use to describe a particular Web page or form may produce valuable information for Web developers.

Much debate has occurred in the library world about tagging and folksonomy, primarily about their flaws. The folksonomy versus taxonomy debate verges into the dogmatic realm much of the time. Proponents of folksonomy argue for the ability of the hive mind and collective intelligence to produce intelligible and findable terms, while taxonomic proponents take one of two stances, either that collective intelligence cannot be trusted to provide accurate or truthful description, or that there are too many semantic problems with folksonomy. For instance, Peterson argues that folksonomies, which can produce contrary or false tags, encourage philosophic relativism and obviate truth, whereas Guy and Tonkin advocate creating smart systems to clean up tags that are "malformed," misspelled, or otherwise questionable.[75,76] The opposition argues that tagging and folksonomies are inherently superior to taxonomies because of high costs associated with taxonomy creation and use, lag time in adding or deleting terms, and because it harnesses collective intelligence.

Though much of the discussion on tagging and folksonomy is thus polarized, many libraries and librarians see value in utilizing both tagging and taxonomies. Several libraries have already begun experimenting with social bookmarking and tagging in OPACs. For instance, Unalog was created by systems librarian Daniel Chudhov; it now serves as a local social bookmarking service for the Yale University School of Medicine.[77] PennTags is another homegrown social bookmarking tool, this one designed by the University of Pennsylvania Library. PennTags, with which users can tag records in the OPAC in addition to Web sites and other materials, is a success; its user base has already added thousands of items to PennTags, including tagging book, music scores, film, and other OPAC records with unique data.[24] Several libraries without their own social bookmarking systems use del.icio.us to either manage

Web site links for use by reference desk staff, or to promote user engagement with the Web site by rolling new links via RSS feeds or by soliciting user link submissions.[78,79] Several libraries incorporate "add to del.icio.us" links into their library Web sites; the Morrisville College Library lets users bookmark directly from the OPAC, for example, and the University of Minnesota Bio-Medical Library puts them on their Web pages. Other libraries and institutions use tagging in their institutional repositories. Library vendors have noticed the tagging trend and are beginning to work on products that will enable users to tag OPAC records. LibraryThing, which was mentioned previously, is one of those vendors; Ex Libris' Primo will be another.

del.icio.us

"that for:user is like the most terse email ever–just the facts, ma'am"
–Jay Datema, personal communication
    Amongst the current social bookmarking tools, del.icio.us is by far the most popular in addition to being the oldest.[80] Though a few tools like Ma.gnolia and BlinkList are considered by some to be better, del.icio.us shines in its simplicity, flexibility, and networking capabilities.[81] One of del.icio.us' major features is Your Network, a way for users to monitor other users' accounts that may be of interest. Indeed, this is one of del.icio.us' most powerful tools, as it creates connection and community amongst its users, plus makes it very easy to stay current with the latest in research, news, and Web resources. One of the networking capabilities is to flag bookmarks for other people by using a special for: syntax (i.e., for:user), a way of sharing Web sites a lot faster and with less annoyance than copying and pasting the URL into an e-mail. Each bookmark on del.icio.us contains information about which users bookmarked it, meaning it is easy to find others with similar interests in del.icio.us.
    Like in MySpace and other social networking sites, people in a del.icio.us network can be total strangers. Unlike in MySpace, being in a network is not so much a form of social capital as it is a practical way to keep on top of what's happening in one's field. This is true for the other social bookmarking tools as well, most especially CiteULike and Connotea, which exist to share data about research publications amongst scholars and scientists. Though most social bookmarking tools allow users to make bookmarks private, public bookmarking is what makes these tools valuable for creating connections and discovering new things.

CONCLUSION

Social networking services comprise a large part of today's Web and show no sign of releasing their hold on the world's psyche any time soon. Libraries can engage their patrons using these tools, whether by connecting with students via Facebook, by posting pertinent Web links in del.icio.us, or helping implement corporate social networking tools.

RESOURCES

All examples and citations used in this paper, plus additional relevant materials, are accessible via Connotea: <http://www.connotea.org/user/ socialsoftware/tag/mrsq-bibliography>.

REFERENCES

1. O'Reilly, T. "What Is Web 2.0: Design Patterns and Business Models for the Next Generation of Software." (September 30, 2005). Available: <http://www. oreillynet.com/ pub/a/oreilly/tim/news/2005/09/30/what-is-web-20.html>. Accessed: October 31, 2006.

2. Allen, C. "Tracing the Evolution of Social Software." *Life with Alacrity.* (October 13, 2004). Available: <http://www.lifewithalacrity.com/2004/10/tracing_the_evo.html>. Accessed: October 31, 2006.

3. Rivlin, G. "Wallflower at the Web Party." *New York Times* (October 15, 2006): 3.1.

4. Alexa Internet Inc. "Top Sites United States." *Top Sites.* (November 1, 2006). Available: <http://www.alexa.com/site/ds/top_sites?cc=US&ts_mode=country&lang=none>. Accessed: November 1, 2006.

5. Alexa Internet Inc. "Top Sites. [Global Top 500]." *Top Sites.* (November 1, 2006). Available: <http://www.alexa.com/site/ds/top_sites?ts_mode=global&lang=none>. Accessed: November 1, 2006.

6. Alexa Internet Inc. "Related Info For: myspace.com." *Traffic Rankings.* (November 1, 2006). Available: <http://www.alexa.com/data/details/traffic_details?url= myspace.com>. Accessed: November 1, 2006.

7. Compete Inc. "myspace.com." *SnapShot.* (November 1, 2006). Available: <http:// snapshot.compete.com/myspace.com>. Accessed: November 1, 2006.

8. Abrams, J.A. "System, Method and Apparatus for Connecting Users in an Online Computer System Based on Their Relationships within Social Networks. United States of America: Friendster, Inc." (2003). Available: <http://patft.uspto.gov/netacgi/ nph-Parser?Sect1=PTO2&Sect2=HITOFF&p=1&u=%2Fnetahtml%2FPTO%2Fsearch-bool.html&r=1&f=G&l=50&co1=AND&d=PTXT&s1=7,069,308.PN.& OS=PN/7,069, 308&RS=PN/7,069,308>. Accessed: October 12, 2006.

9. Sjoberg, L. "MySpace, Now with Random Crap." *Wired News* (October 25, 2006). Available: <http://www.wired.com/news/columns/0,71998-0.html>. Accessed: November 11, 2006.

10. boyd, d. 2006. "Identity Production in a Networked Culture: Why Youth Heart MySpace." Paper presented at American Association for the Advancement of Science, February 19, at St. Louis, MO.

11. Vincent, F. "MySpace for Musicians." *Electronic Musician.* (July 1, 2006). Available: <http://emusician.com/tutorials/emusic_myspace_musicians/>. Accessed: November 11, 2006.

12. Levy, S., and Stone, B. "The New Wisdom of the Web." *Newsweek* (April 3, 2006): 46-53.

13. Russell, M. 2006. "myspace for Thousands." *Post-Bulletin* (April 11, 2006): A1, A6.

14. Garrett, J.J. "MySpace: Design Anarchy That Works." *Business Week Online* (January 3, 2006): 16.

15. House of Representatives. *Deleting Online Predators Act.* 109th Congress, H.R. 5319, 2006.

16. American Library Association. "DOPA." (2006). Available: <http://www.ala.org/ala/washoff/WOissues/techinttele/dopa/DOPA.htm>. Accessed: November 14, 2006.

17. Young Adult Library Services Association. "Social Networking and DOPA." *YALSA Blog* (November 2, 2006). Available: <http://www.leonline.com/yalsa/positive_uses.pdf>. Accessed: November 14, 2006.

18. NJIT Library Research Desk. "Be in Our Top 8!–Students/Alumni Only!" *NJIT Library Research Desk MySpace Blog* (October 12, 2006). Available: <http://blog.myspace.com/index.cfm?fuseaction=blog.view&friendID=82376801&blogID=179649880>. Accessed: November 14, 2006.

19. Evans, B. "Your Space or MySpace?" *Library Journal netConnect* (October 15, 2006): 8-12.

20. Noguchi, Y. "In Teens' Web World, MySpace Is So Last Year; Social Sites Find Fickle Audience." *Washington Post* (October 29, 2006): A.1.

21. Vara, V. "MySpace, ByeSpace?; Some Users Renounce Social Sites as Too Big." *Wall Street Journal* (October 26, 2006): B.1.

22. Stutzman, F. "What Comscore's Traffic Numbers Really Mean." *Unit Structures.* (October 21, 2006). Available: <http://chimprawk.blogspot.com/2006/10/what-comscores-traffic-numbers-really.html>. Accessed: November 14, 2006.

23. Prescott, L. "Social Networking Sites Recover from September Decline, Facebook Visits up 16%." *Hitwise Intelligence Analyst Blogs* (November 8, 2006). Available: <http://weblogs.hitwise.com/leeann-prescott/2006/11/social_networking_sites_recove.html>. Accessed: November 14, 2006.

24. Medical Library Association. Moving at the Speed of Byte: Emerging Technologies for Information Management: College of DuPage. (2006).

25. Dr. Date [pseud.]. "Dear Logged Off, Dr. Date." *The Minnesota Daily* (November 13, 2006): 9B.

26. Stutzman, F. "Facebook Is Now Open, but Is It Relevant?" *Unit Structures.* (September 26, 2006). Available: <http://chimprawk.blogspot.com/2006/09/ facebook-is-now-open-but-is-it.html>. Accessed: November 15, 2006.

27. Stutzman, F. "Student Life on the Facebook." *Unit Structures.* (January 8, 2006). Available: <http://chimprawk.blogspot.com/2006/01/student-life-on-facebook.html>. Accessed: November 15, 2006.

28. Stutzman, F. "Adopting the Facebook: A Comparative Analysis." *Unit Structures.* (July 7, 2006). Available: <http://chimprawk.blogspot.com/2006/07/adopting-facebook-comparative-analysis.html>. Accessed: November 15, 2006.

29. Vanden Bogaart, M.R. *Uncovering the Social Impacts of Facebook on a College Campus.* (Masters thesis). Manhattan, KS: Department of Counseling and Educational Psychology, College of Education, Kansas State University, 2006.

30. Yadav, S., and Cashmore, P. "Facebook–the Complete Biography." *Mashable* (August 25, 2006). Available: <http://mashable.com/2006/08/25/facebook-profile/>. Accessed: November 3, 2006.

31. Bugeja, M.J. "Facing the Facebook." *Chronicle of Higher Education* (January 27, 2006): C1-C4.

32. Stutzman, F. "Situational Relevance in Social Networking Websites." *Unit Structures.* (January 12, 2006). Available: <http://chimprawk.blogspot.com/2006/01/situational-relevance-in-social.html>. Accessed: November 3, 2006.

33. Stutzman, F. "Facebook: A Generation's Identity Archive." *Unit Structures* (September 5, 2006). Available: <http://chimprawk.blogspot.com/2006/09/facebook-generations-identity-archive.html>. Accessed: November 15, 2006.

34. Schneier, B. "Lessons from the Facebook Riots." *Wired News* (September 21, 2006). Available: <http://www.wired.com/news/columns/0,71815-0.html>. Accessed: November 15, 2006.

35. Snider, M. 2006. "iPods Knock over Beer Mugs ; College Kids Rank What's Most Popular." *USA TODAY* (June 8, 2006): D.9.

36. Mathews, B.S. "Do You Facebook?" *College & Research Libraries News* 67, no. 5 (2006): 306-7.

37. Mathews, B.S. "Welcoming Freshmen: CeLIBration @ the GT Library PART 1 (Intro/Concept)." *Ubiquitous Librarian* (August 21, 2006). Available: <http://theubiquitouslibrarian.typepad.com/the_ubiquitous_librarian/2006/08/welcoming_fresh.html>. Accessed: November 15, 2006.

38. Mathews, B.S. "[Ubiquitous Librarian Posts Tagged CeLIBration]." *Ubiquitous Librarian* (September 14, 2006). Available: <http://theubiquitouslibrarian.typepad.com/the_ubiquitous_librarian/celibration/index.html>. Accessed: November 15, 2006.

39. Mathews, B.S. "Games @ the GT Library (CeLIBration, PART 4)." *Ubiquitous Librarian* (August 30, 2006). Available: <http://theubiquitouslibrarian.typepad.com/the_ubiquitous_librarian/2006/08/games_the_gt_li.html>. Accessed: November 15, 2006.

40. Farkas, M. "Facebook at Bennington's Crossett Library." *Information Wants To Be Free.* (May 22, 2006). Available: <http://meredith.wolfwater.com/wordpress/index.php/2006/05/22/facebook-at-benningtons-crossett-library/>. Accessed: November 15, 2006.

41. Drew, W. "FaceBook Closing Organization Pages Such as Libraries." *Baby Boomer Librarian* (August 25, 2006). Available: <http://babyboomerlibrarian.blogspot.com/2006/08/facebook-closing-organization-pages.html>. Accessed: November 15, 2006.

42. Kraemer, B. "Facebook Account." *Web4lib* (October 25, 2006). Available: <http://lists.webjunction.org/wjlists/web4lib/2006-October/041984.html>. Accessed: November 15, 2006.

43. Stutzman, F. "Facebook Is Killing the Fakesters." *Unit Structures* (September 25, 2006). Available: <http://chimprawk.blogspot.com/2006/09/facebook-is-killing-fakesters.html>. Accessed: November 15, 2006.

44. Mathews, B.S. "What to Do When Facebook Closes Down Your Library Storefront." *Ubiquitous Librarian* (October 4, 2006). Available: <http://theubiquitous

librarian.typepad.com/the_ubiquitous_librarian/2006/10/what_to_do_when.html>. Accessed: November 16, 2006.

45. The EDUCAUSE Learning Initiative. "7 Things You Should Know About Facebook." *7 Things* (2006). Available: <http://www.educause.edu/ir/library/pdf/ELI7017.pdf>. Accessed: November 16, 2006.

46. Trapani, G. "Friends List." *Scribbling.net* (July 29, 2006). Available: <http://scribbling.net/friends-list>. Accessed: November 16, 2006.

47. Bruce, C. "Six Apart Leads with Vox." *Wired News* (November 7, 2006). Available: <http://www.wired.com/news/technology/internet/0,72072-0.html>. Accessed: November 15, 2006.

48. Iskold, A., and MacManus, R. "The Social Networking Faceoff." *Read/Write Web* (September 21, 2006). Available: <http://www.readwriteweb.com/archives/social_network_faceoff.php>. Accessed: November 17, 2006.

49. Richardson, W. "New Tools for Edbloggers." *weblogg-ed* (October 28, 2006). Available: <http://weblogg-ed.com/2006/new-tools-for-edbloggers/>. Accessed: November 15, 2006.

50. Zobitz, P.; Rethlefsen, M.; Segovis, C. et al. "Social Networking Goes to Medical School: The Creation of an Online Community to Facilitate Faculty-Student Interaction." Paper presented at E-Learn 2006, October 14, 2006, Honolulu, HI.

51. Tosh, D., and Werdmuller, B. "Creation of a Learning Landscape: Webblogging and Social Networking in the Context of E-Portfolios." (July 15, 2004). Available: <http://eradc.org/papers/Learning_landscape.pdf>. Accessed: November 15, 2006.

52. Berry, M. "Elgg and Blogging in Primary Education." (January 2006). Available: <http://elgg.net/mberry/files/-1/3567/primary_blogging.pdf>. Accessed: November 15, 2006.

53. Stanier, S. "1000 Posts. Implementing Elgg in H.E." (November 15, 2006). Available: <http://elgg.net/impelgg/weblog/139101.html>. Accessed: November 15, 2006.

54. Anderson, T. "Distance Learning–Social Software's Killer Ap?" Paper presented at 17th Biennial Conference of the Open and Distance Learning Association of Australia, 2006, Adelaide, South Australia.

55. Gittlen, S. "An Open Source Education." *Network World* (September 25, 2006). Available: <http://www.networkworld.com/allstar/2006/092506-open-source-saugus-union-school-district.html>. Accessed: November 17, 2006.

56. Fried, I. "Gates Demonstrates New Search Software." *CNET*. (May 17, 2006). Available: <http://news.com.com/2100-1012_3-6073028.html>. Accessed: November 15, 2006.

57. Writer, B.G.I.B. "Corporate America Embraces Social Networking." *Oakland Tribune* (October 16, 2006): 1.

58. Farrell, S., and Lau, T. "Fringe Contacts: People-Tagging for the Enterprise." Paper presented at WWW2006 Collaborative Tagging Workshop, May 22, 2006, Edinburgh, Scotland.

59. Ezzy, E., and MacManus, R. "Social Networking: Time for a Silver Bullet." *Read/Write Web*. (October 4, 2006). Available: <http://www.readwriteweb.com/archives/social_networking_silver_bullet.php>. Accessed: November 20, 2006.

60. Stutzman, F. "Del.icio.us Is Already a Social Network." *Unit Structures*. (October 5, 2006). Available: <http://chimprawk.blogspot.com/2006/10/delicious-is-already-social-network.html>. Accessed: November 21, 2006.

61. Sherman, C. "Hacking Flickr." *Search Engine Watch.* (June 21, 2006). Available: <http://searchenginewatch.com/showPage.html?page=3614881>. Accessed: November 18, 2006.

62. Stephens, M. "Steal This Idea: Flickr for Librarians." *Tame the Web.* (September 18, 2006). Available: <http://www.tametheweb.com/2006/09/steal_this_idea_flickr_for_lib.html>. Accessed: November 20, 2006.

63. Saunders, J. "Flickr as a Digital Collection Host." *SLAIS to CLA Conference* (August 22, 2006). Available: <http://slaistocla.blogspot.com/2006/08/flickr-as-digital-collection-host.html>. Accessed: November 20, 2006.

64. Danigirl. "That Library Thing." *Postcards from the Mothership.* (October 5, 2005). Available: <http://momm-eh.blogspot.com/2005/10/that-library-thing.html>. Accessed: November 20, 2006.

65. Rethlefsen, M.L. "Product Pipeline. Melissa L. Rethlefesen Looks at Book-Sharing Sites and iPod Reference Content and What They Mean to Librarians." *Library Journal netConnect* (January 15, 2007): 14-6.

66. Rethlefsen, M.L. "Chief Thingamabrian: LJ talks to Tim Spalding." *Library Journal* 132, no. 1 (2007): 40-2.

67. Grossman, L. "Best Invention. YouTube." *TIME Best Inventions 2006.* (2006). Available: <http://www.time.com/time/2006/techguide/bestinventions/inventions/youtube.html>. Accessed: November 20, 2006.

68. The EDUCAUSE Learning Initiative. "7 Things You Should Know About YouTube." *7 Things.* (September, 2006). Available: <http://www.educause.edu/LibraryDetailPage/666?ID=ELI7018>. Accessed: November 20, 2006.

69. Rethlefsen, M.L. "Product Pipeline. Melissa L. Rethlefsen Looks at Social Reference Managers and What They Mean for Librarians." *Library Journal netConnect* (October 15, 2006): 14-6.

70. Rethlefsen, M.L. "Product Pipeline. Melissa L. Rethlefsen Looks at Social Bookmarking Services and What They Mean to Librarians." *Library Journal netConnect* (July 15, 2006): 16-7.

71. Johnston, P. "dctagging." *eFoundations.* (October 8, 2006). Available: <http://efoundations.typepad.com/efoundations/2006/10/dctagged.html>. Accessed: November 21, 2006.

72. Orchard, L.M. "Tagging Hacks." In *Hacking del.icio.us,* edited by L. M. Orchard. Indianapolis, IN: Wiley Publishing, Inc., 2006

73. Golder, S., and Huberman, B.A. "The Structure of Collaborative Tagging Systems." arXiv.org. (August 15, 2005). Available: <http://arxiv.org/pdf/cs.DL/0508082>. Accessed: November 19, 2006.

74. Millen, D.; Feinberg, J.; and Kerr, B. "Social Bookmarking in the Enterprise." *Social Computing* 3, no. 9 (2005). Available: <http://acmqueue.com/modules.php?name=Content&pa=showpage&pid=344>. Accessed: November 21, 2006.

75. Peterson, E. 2006. "Beneath the Metadata: Some Philosophical Problems with Folksonomy." *D-Lib Magazine* 12, no. 11 (2006). Available: <http://www.dlib.org/dlib/november06/peterson/11peterson.html>. Accessed: November 21, 2006.

76. Guy, M., and Tonkin, E. "Folksonomies: Tidying up Tags?" *D-Lib Magazine* 11, no. 1 (2006). Available: <http://www.dlib.org/dlib/january06/guy/01guy.html>. Accessed: November 21, 2006.

77. Chudnov, D.; Barnett, J.; Prasad, R.; and Wilcox, M. "Experiments in Academic Social Book Marking with Unalog." *Library Hi Tech* 23, no. 4 (2005): 469-80.

78. Etches-Johnson, A. "Delicious, Indeed." *Blog Without a Library* (July 13, 2006). Available: <http://www.blogwithoutalibrary.net/?p=213>. Accessed: November 21, 2006.

79. Rethlefsen, M.L.; Engard, N.C.; Chang, D.; and Haytko, C. "Social Software for Libraries and Librarians." *Journal of Hospital Librarianship* 6, no. 4 (2006): 29-45.

80. Iskold, A., and MacManus, R. "The Social Bookmarking Faceoff." *Read/Write Web*. (September 18, 2006). Available: <http://www.readwriteweb.com/archives/social_bookmarking_faceoff.php>. Accessed: November 21, 2006.

81. Gilbertson, S. "Social Bookmarking Showdown." *Wired News* (November 6, 2006). Available: <http://www.wired.com/news/technology/internet/1,72070-0.html>. Accessed: November 21, 2006.

doi:10.1300/J115v26S01_07

Content Management
and Web 2.0 with Drupal

Chad M. Fennell

SUMMARY. The University of Minnesota Health Sciences Libraries undertook several major Web-related projects in 2006, including a complete overhaul of those systems supporting Web content publishing at the libraries. Based upon identified user needs and internal technology support considerations, the Health Sciences Libraries chose a popular open source content management tool known as "Drupal." This paper discusses content management system components and how they are manifested in the Drupal framework. The Health Sciences Libraries' local installation is then considered in more detail. doi:10.1300/J115v26S01_08 *[Article copies available for a fee from The Haworth Document Delivery Service: 1-800-HAWORTH. E-mail address: <docdelivery@haworthpress.com> Website: <http://www. HaworthPress.com> © 2007 by The Haworth Press, Inc. All rights reserved.]*

KEYWORDS. Content management systems, CMS, Drupal, open source software, OSS

Chad M. Fennell, MSLS (fenne035@umn.edu) is a Web Developer and Health Informatics Specialist, University of Minnesota Health Sciences Libraries, Bio-Medical Library, Diehl Hall, 505 Essex Street SE, Minneapolis, MN 55455-0334. He holds a B.A in English Literature and an M.S. in Library Science from the University of Illinois at Urbana-Champaign.

[Haworth co-indexing entry note]: "Content Management and Web 2.0 with Drupal." Fennell, Chad M. Co-published simultaneously in *Medical Reference Services Quarterly* (The Haworth Information Press, an imprint of The Haworth Press, Inc.) Vol. 26, Supp. #1, 2007, pp. 143-167; and: *Medical Librarian 2.0: Use of Web 2.0 Technologies in Reference Services* (ed: M. Sandra Wood) The Haworth Information Press, an imprint of The Haworth Press, Inc., 2007, pp. 143-167. Single or multiple copies of this article are available for a fee from The Haworth Document Delivery Service [1-800-HAWORTH, 9:00 a.m. - 5:00 p.m. (EST). E-mail address: docdelivery@haworthpress.com].

Available online at http://mrsq.haworthpress.com
© 2007 by The Haworth Press, Inc. All rights reserved.
doi:10.1300/J115v26S01_08

INTRODUCTION

As libraries move forward, many will likely be forced to address greater volumes of Web content and increased clamoring for more participation in the Web presence on the part of library staff. Others may see a rise in the demand for more highly personalized services for end users.[1,2] It therefore seems natural that many libraries would find their way to the concept of "Web content management." However, learning about this practice is only the first step in a very long journey.

A cursory glance at the seemingly innumerable options in the area of Web content management (WCM), and it is hard to fault library Web committees and library technologists for throwing up their collective hands at the host of options. One is forced to compare radically different types of systems, fundamentally differing approaches, and inconsistent terminology and match all this with organizational needs. Even the basic labels for content management seem to vary widely: Web content management (WCM), enterprise content management (ECM), Web enterprise content management (WECM), content management system (CMS), etc. As a first step towards clarification, the initialism "CMS" will serve as the primary name for "Web content management" in the context of this discussion.

This paper addresses issues surrounding the motivation for moving to a content management system, a description of core CMS components (with comparisons to the current system at the Health Sciences Libraries), and a discussion of the Health Sciences Libraries' (HSL) implementation of a content management tool known as "Drupal." The Health Sciences Libraries has successfully implemented Drupal and continues to develop new features in order to meet user needs.

WHY MOVE TO A CONTENT MANAGEMENT SYSTEM?

Reasons for moving to a content management system vary from organization to organization. Holly Yu in *Library Web Content Management: Needs and Challenges* identifies a number of common considerations: a growth in the demand for personalization on the part of users; the need to put new forms of content, such as calendars, online; increased size and complexity of library sites, and more.[1] Robert Boiko, in his *Content Management Bible,* suggests four principle motivating factors for moving to a CMS: too much content, too many contributors, too much change, or too many publications.[2] It's also important to recognize just how much content size will continue to grow in the future and to find ways to accommodate increased demands for access.[3] If a library is struggling with any of these issues, a content management solution may be in order. Often there is resistance from library webmasters, who are struggling to keep site content up to date while performing a wide variety of other tasks. Content management systems are attractive to libraries because they offer the possibility of streamlining content maintenance, improving content re-use, standardizing output, and generally reducing the cost of managing content that would otherwise be highly labor intensive.[1]

The Health Sciences Libraries moved to a content management solution for several key reasons: to improve staff access to, and hence ownership over, the library Web presence; to streamline the management of repetitive and recurring content such as staff contact lists, library events, and library workshop postings; and to generally provide an enhanced toolkit for the provision of online library services. Until the Health Sciences Libraries implemented Drupal, content was managed on the older "webmaster" model, where changes were submitted to a webmaster, who then made all direct changes to the site. An improved mechanism for handling content would help the libraries to effectively leverage more staff for the purpose of Web page management and to generally position the library to do more with its Web presence.

WHAT ARE CONTENT MANAGEMENT SYSTEMS?

Drawing heavily upon Robert Boiko's *Content Management Bible,* a framework for understanding Web content management first and then examining Drupal as a Web content management system second will be presented. Content management is discussed here from two basic perspectives: basic architectural considerations and what a CMS does.

Basic Architectural Considerations for a CMS

While there is certainly no one single definition of what a CMS is, many have at least acknowledged the wide confusion between content management tools and content management systems, both inside and outside of the library community.[1,2] The online library environment is characterized by a diverse range of applications and content-bearing utilities that must work together to produce a library Web presence. Any successful content management system must be able to effectively bind these tools and services together; but, such tools or a collection of such tools do not necessarily constitute a content management system. A library may, for example, provide an automated means of delivering online pathfinders for subject specialists, which is a mechanism for managing online content but does not represent a full CMS.[4] Libraries also often employ Web authoring tools such as Dreamweaver or Microsoft Front Page to manage their Web content. These tools also do not qualify as content management systems as they do not provide many of the core features of a full CMS, such as a centralized metadata framework.

There is also wide confusion between full content management systems and mere "dynamic Web sites."[1,2,4] Dynamic sites pull content from a data source such as a database, transform the content into HTML, and serve this HTML to end users. Static sites, on the other hand, are simply a collection of HTML files. A full content management system has the capability to generate static file and dynamically rendered sites, providing architectures for both models as well as for mixed models where some content is static and some dynamic.[2] Additionally, a CMS can typically render content into non-Web formats, setting it apart from a simple dynamic site model where Web output is the only option.[2] Still, as the discussion turns towards typical CMS features, it will become clear that, to some extent, the label of "content management system" is more a matter of degree than an absolute identity.

In thinking about content management strategies available within full content management systems, Boiko characterizes these as falling into essentially two basic varieties: "modular" or "linear."[2] "Modular" systems break down content into distinct units or "chunks" that bear a weak cross-content relationship (units are relatively unconnected with other units), whereas "Linear" systems situate highly granular content units (usually nested between and labeled by XML tags) into an overarching hierarchy, a kind of tightly woven narrative.[2]

Linear systems better address the needs of sites that present content with a strong central narrative, such as online books where components such as paragraphs fit into organizational units like book chapters.[2] Due to the capability of linear systems to label content in this highly granular fashion, they allow for the maximum level of content re-use.[2] This fact results from the ability of such a system to search for and manipulate content that has been labeled or "marked up" with XML tags, which contain descriptive information about the given item.[2] For example, if each time content was added to such a system authors were required to label the names of people with the appropriate XML (or other markup system) tag, one could easily create an index of names by searching the content repository and harvesting all content with this tag.

Modular systems generally break content into small "chunks," which are often stored in a database, and rely upon associated metadata to repurpose these chunks into various portions of a site.[2] The focus of a strictly modular system is upon manipulating content at the "chunk" level. This kind of arrangement is well suited to the needs of organization sites where content with weak cross-content relationships exist, such as with FAQs, press releases, events, job postings, downloads, or workshops predominate. Here, describing information at the "chunk" level allows for sufficient repurposing and manipulation of site content. Generally speaking, modular systems offer slightly less descriptive power but also a lower maintenance overhead in terms of this description.

While Drupal likely does not technically meet the definition of a full Web content management system, it possesses a great number of the hallmarks of such systems, much more so than many other dynamic site systems. Drupal, for example, resembles a modular content management system as described above in that metadata is associated with chunks of content in the form of a site taxonomy and in that the CMS serves content associated with this metadata as its core content re-use strategy. Content chunks are comprised of a set of information that is stored in a relational database as a set of associated tables. Information that makes up each chunk includes, but is not limited to, a title, a body, a "content type" designator (e.g., "news feature"), a version history, an author/contributor id, a publication status (e.g., published, unpublished), a creation date/time, a modification date/time, a comment log, access and permissions settings, and statistical tracking information. Drupal combines this set of information with a centralized taxonomy system to realize the functionality of a modular system. Developers and administrators have a variety of options for manipulating chunks of content, especially by querying the Drupal content repository (i.e., the database) for items associated with terms from a given taxonomy. Drupal offers a number of default mechanisms for retrieving content associated with site taxonomy items. Site taxonomy terms may be, for example, easily displayed next to each content chunk. Those familiar with blogs will find features such as these familiar. Here, when a user clicks on a taxonomy term, all content associated with the given term will be dynamically queried and rendered to the page. This is but one example of what may be done with the simple taxonomy/content chunk model that Drupal provides. Developers will find many ways to build upon this framework so as to maximize content re-use and content value more generally.

WHAT A CMS DOES

Among the many difficulties of describing and discussing content management systems, the problem of identifying core system functions common to all content management systems is among the most difficult. It is, however, often easier to understand content management systems by "what they do" rather than by the more abstract discussion of "what they are" (e.g., modular vs. linear). If it looks like a content management system, it may be a content management system. Robert Boiko outlines three basic functions of a CMS: the collection, management, and publication of content.[2] These three aspects encompass the entire life-cycle of content within such systems and provide a high-level framework for discussing CMS features.

Content Collection as an Aspect of a CMS

First in the process of content management comes content collection. Here, data is gathered into the CMS. Boiko subdivides content collection into five aspects: authoring, acquisition, conversion, aggregation, and collection services.[2] Here, "authoring" simply refers to the process of generating new content "from scratch."[2] Acquisition then refers to the gathering of external content into the system. Conversion occurs as unwanted information (e.g., unwanted HTML tags) or data is filtered out from the wanted data or information in a give piece of content. Boiko defines "aggregation" as to "edit the content, divide it into components, and augment it to fit within your desired metadata system."[2] Finally, "collection services" are "programs and functions that aid the collection process," such as Web forms.[2] Because these definitions are essentially generic abstractions of general practices in content management, there will be cases where the lines between processes blur and exceptions must be made. Content conversion, for example, is essentially a part of both the authoring and acquisition processes.[2] Still, Boiko offers a relatively stable set of high-level concepts with which to investigate content management system design.

Turning to Drupal's content collection features, "authoring" content is by far the dominant path for content uptake into the system. In the authoring phase of content management, Drupal provides quite similar functionality to fully-fledged content management systems. The basic architecture of the system also allows for significant modification of authoring interfaces as well as for the introduction of new functionalities to augment the process, for example. Boiko outlines a number of core features typical of the authoring components of a CMS: the provision of an authoring environment; interfaces to promote the authoring of audience-specific content; the provision of various authoring aides; the existence of templates and forms to break down content into its core components for editing; and the existence of workflow, content status (published, unpublished, etc.) and content version control features.[2] Fundamentally, these features enhance the ability of authors to contribute content while also providing managers and administrators with mechanisms to assure the quality of content as it comes into the system. Drupal possesses all of these features in some measure.

The authoring environment and collection system of Drupal exists within the context of the Web site. That is to say, Drupal channels the content authoring process primarily through Web forms, although other options, such as contribution by e-mail, do exist as add-on features. And, as with many content management systems, Drupal provides mechanisms to facilitate authoring, such as the automatic recording of author and date information. Upon logging into Drupal, content contributors (authors) will notice a menu appear for content authoring (see Figure 1).

FIGURE 1. Content Types

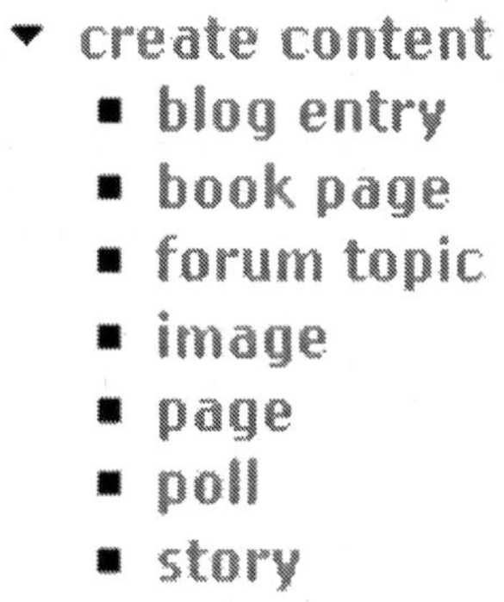

- ▼ create content
  - ■ blog entry
  - ■ book page
  - ■ forum topic
  - ■ image
  - ■ page
  - ■ poll
  - ■ story

Like many content management systems, Drupal utilizes the concept of "content types." In Drupal, these are called "node types," although content contributors will likely never need to know this terminology. Content types (node types) in Drupal represent the basic forms of content that may be created by system users. Each type is constructed in such a way that it provides specialized content collection interfaces and functionalities, including the ability to provide content type-specific template styles. Content contributors, however, will simply understand that they can create different kinds of content, depending upon the need at hand. Drupal comes bundled with a few standard content types, but many other content types exist as installable modules. Site administrators can easily install and configure these additional content types. Content types available for installation by site administrators allow users, for example, to make their own polls for others to vote on, create e-mail contact forms, upload images and auto-generate thumbnail and previews versions, post forum topics, and more. The content types displayed in Figure 1 represent those that come with Drupal (e.g., "page") as well as several add-on content types (e.g., "story). After selecting a content type to create, Drupal users will then be presented with a content form (see Figure 2).

With Drupal 4.7, the submission forms have seen significant usability improvement. Using "gracefully degrading" javascript practice (i.e., writing Javascript that merely enhances the visual interface but which will not cause the process to fail if Javascript is turned off on the end user's browser), Drupal developers made all form menu and features collapsible. Further, text boxes are enhanced with Javascript in that their size is easily adjusted by clicking on and dragging a bar located at the bottom of each box. There are a number of other Javascript-specific enhancements as well.

FIGURE 2. Content Submission Form

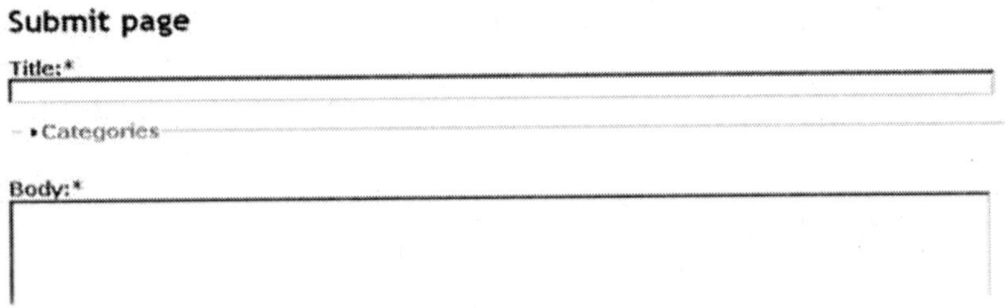

Submit page

Title:*

▸Categories

Body:*

Boiko also indicates workflow, status, and version control as components of authoring systems, although such features are also administered centrally as part of the management system.[2] A workflow is, simply, a set of states or phases that some content must go through on the way to publication. A common use for a workflow in a content management system is to incorporate levels of review into the publication of the content. For example, many organizations require a content editor and/or a webmaster to review contributions for style, both in terms of appearance and tone of the content. Workflows help in this process by sending out e-mails to the appropriate parties and moving the content to various states as approvals or recommendations are given by reviewers. Formal workflows in Drupal exist as an add-on module (i.e., the "workflow" module) and are not mature relative to larger, more enterprise-level systems. Workflows in Drupal are in a state of active development and will likely mature in upcoming versions. Content status and revision are, however, well supported Drupal features. The status of any given item of content in Drupal can be either "published" or "unpublished," which determines whether or not end users can see it. Unpublished drafts of current pages are also possible as of Drupal 4.7 and look to become part of Drupal's core offerings in upcoming versions.[5] Version control in Drupal allows users to view old versions of a given piece of content and to roll content back to this original version. Modules also exist to enhance this functionality, such as adding the ability to highlight differences between versions with color and text strikethroughs.

Acquisition features are fairly weak in Drupal, involving only the importing of content from other Drupal instances or via custom-written modules for other sources. However, because of Drupal's relatively simple architecture and support for Web services, building custom import scripts would be a reasonably approachable task for most developers. More "robust" acquisition features might include such items as drag and drop file folder import capability or mass import tools for the migration of one content management system to another.

Drupal largely does not provide mechanisms for transforming content from one format to another. More robust enterprise-level content management systems provide such mechanisms.[2] This is one area where Drupal acts more as a simple Web content management "tool" than a "complete" content management system. Drupal does have limited but highly useful capabilities where images are concerned. The "Image" module allows system administrators to configure Drupal to automatically produce three separate image sizes on the fly: "thumbnail," "preview," and "original." The thumbnail and preview versions are produced on the server, and the system can be configured to produce images of specific dimensions.

Drupal also offers a number of mechanisms for aggregating content. As mentioned earlier, Drupal comes with a taxonomy system. The Drupal taxonomy system allows for nested taxonomies called "Vocabularies." Vocabularies are associated with content types by administrators who determine which content types will have access to a given vocabulary. Site administrators may, for example, create a "News" vocabulary that only appears in news content creation and editing forms. Content contributors, therefore, only see those portions of the site taxonomy that pertain to their given content task and are not bombarded with a great deal of non-relevant terms.

Content Management as an Aspect of a CMS

The second aspect of Boiko's three part division of content management deals with the "management" of content. He outlines four primary components of the management system: a repository, system administration, workflow, and connections.[2] CMS Repositories often involve a variety of data sources from databases to file systems that house the content as well as the configuration data for the system.[2] Often, the content is stored both within a database and as flat files within a file system where file types, such as PDFs, are more highly accessible.[2] Another common approach in enterprise content management is to store Web content in flat files as XML with configuration and metadata in a database. A wide variety of combinations of such approaches are, in fact, possible. Administration systems provide the ability to configure and control all aspects of the CMS. Workflow modules provide a CMS with the facility to control work processes. Notice that while workflows exist in authoring areas of a CMS, they also may exist in other areas, for example, to facilitate system maintenance tasks.[2] Finally, connection services provide a CMS with the ability to connect to information sources outside of the system itself, as with a human resources employee information management system.[2]

Drupal offers all four of these features: a repository, an administrative interface, workflow, and connections, although both workflow and connections are relatively weak in Drupal. In looking at enterprise content management, all four areas are relatively "light" in terms of feature sets and robustness; however, for the purposes of basic Web content management, Drupal offers a powerful, if somewhat limited, feature set.

Drupal's administrative features offer a glimpse into the power that the system offers. Drupal presents robust site template and theme capabilities, role-based user access management, a centralized taxonomy creation and maintenance system, statistical tracking for both errors and user-system interactions, orphan page identification (orphan pages are Web pages that have no "parent" page within the navigation system), system functionality management, and much more. A central element of the Drupal administrative interface and architecture is the concept of Drupal "modules." The module system is a standardized framework for adding to and extending Drupal functionality. Third-party modules may be downloaded from the Drupal Web site and now automatically installed from the administrative interface. With Drupal 4.7, the system also automatically installs all related database tables and offers mechanisms to prevent issues with related modules, such as where one module relies upon another to fully function. Support for these modules, it should be noted, is inconsistent, and care should be taken to verify the status of a given module where a site will depend on its use. A more detailed discussion of all of these features is perhaps out of scope for this discussion, but a more in-depth examination of those most relevant to the Health Sciences Libraries will occur as the discussion turns towards an examination of the Libraries' local installation.

While there is always an "administration area" to each Drupal installation, the look and feel of this site section is determined by the styles and templates established by the site administrator. That is to say, there is no "standard" look to the administration area for Drupal. This approach offers a great deal of flexibility to site administrators and designers in shaping the look and feel of every aspect of the system. However, after the initial installation, users often find administration features somewhat lacking in clarity in terms of providing an obvious path for site administration. There exists a general acknowledgement of this issue and a Drupal usability user group has developed to address it. Another effort that will help to mitigate the problem for new site administrators is the automated installation process that is currently in development, which will come bundled as a standard feature of Drupal in the future. This tool will allow for "standard installations" and will provide an installation "wizard," eliminating the need for site administrators to individually select and install Drupal features. Distributions initially will be geared towards popular configuration options and will be centered around popular themes such as "community sites," "brochure sites," or "corporate sites." Further, organizations and development firms will be able to create their own custom distributions of Drupal as well. It is hoped that these efforts will begin to flatten the initial learning curve for site administration.

Workflow and connections to outside data sources in Drupal, as discussed previously, are relatively weak. Workflow, for example, is non-existent where system administration tasks are concerned. Steps for database backups, user management processes, etc., must be handled manually by systems administrators. Connections to outside data sources in Drupal are feasible with Drupal's XML Web services utilities, but these features are also immature. Web developers could certainly connect outside data sources to Drupal, but this is not a core strength of the system. In considering these "shortcomings," it is also important to recognize the limited scope of target functionality as an exclusively dynamic Web content system. Robust workflows for administrative tasks, for example, make less sense for such a small system.

Content Publication as an Aspect of a CMS

After content collection and management comes the actual publishing portion of a CMS. The publishing system is responsible for "pulling content components and other resources out of the repository and automatically creating publications out of them."[2] Often times, it is the publication management capabilities that draw organizations to content management systems as administrators and Web professionals seek to standardize the "look and feel" of a library Web presence. To accomplish the standardization of output, content management systems employ template systems where content is inserted into a pre-built framework of HTML. The publication system also manages how content is retrieved and inserted into these templates. By controlling what information is gathered and how it is presented, the publication system provides total control over the output of a CMS.

Drupal offers a powerful set of interfaces for controlling both templates and the content gathered into them. The combination of Drupal's themes system and Block Module allows Drupal to present highly granular control over content output in the system. The theme system of Drupal consists of a template rendering utility (a "template engine") as well as the actual templates. It allows site administrators to install, develop, and enable site template themes. This functionality extends down to the individual user level as administrators can enable multiple themes for any given site and allow users to override the default theme (see Figure 3), giving them the power to change the site appearance for their own use.

FIGURE 3. User Theme Configuration

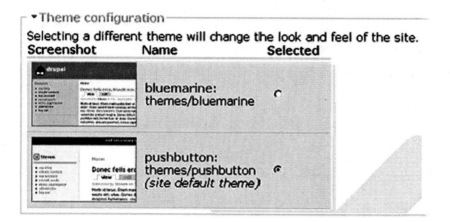

In the library setting, this feature could provide an interesting mechanism for the creation of more highly accessible sites where an "accessibility template" option might be presented to users as an alternate Drupal theme. Themes consist of a set of templates to control the various types of content on a given site. One of the key benefits to building new content types in Drupal is that it allows developers to also build a template for each content type. Library staff contact pages, for example, could have a completely different layout than other sorts of pages on the site. Another strength of the Drupal template system is that it makes heavy use of Cascading Style Sheets (CSS) design techniques where virtually every element created by Drupal can be styled using CSS. The bias towards CSS design means Drupal is in step with current trends in Web design and will be all the more attractive to library Web designers as a result.

Another powerful feature of Drupal's theme system is that of "content regions." Content regions consist of an unlimited number of configurable areas where content may appear in a given template. Templates will automatically provide regions for the main content, a header area, a footer area, a right sidebar area, and a left sidebar area. Administrators and developers can push content into these regions within a given template and even make their own custom regions. Within a template, regions appear as snippets of code that developers place in areas of the template where they would like the dynamic content to appear. As the publication system processes the page, it replaces the code snippets (the regions) with the appropriate content for that region. To get a full understanding of content regions, a discussion of "content blocks" in Drupal is in order.

"Blocks" in Drupal are simply chunks of content that can be inserted into content regions on a given template. Fortunately for the "code-challenged," Drupal provides a graphical interface to configure where content blocks will appear (see Figure 4) within a given template.

Content for blocks can be generated "behind the scenes" from a Drupal module or manually by creating a content block directly through the blocks menu. An example of a block generated by a module external to the Block Module is the "User Login" block, which is generated by the User Module. The User Module handles user management in Drupal and creates a small block of HTML content for a login form. Then, in the Blocks menu, site administrators can determine in which region in the template this user login form will appear. But there is more to block configuration than determining where in a template it can appear. Several more configuration options exist. A block also has a "weight." The weight of a given block determines where it will appear in relation to other blocks in the respective template region. If a block has a low weight number, it is "light" and will "float" to the top of the list and appear above other "heavier" blocks. Essentially, administrators are simply adjusting the sorting order of the output of blocks in adjusting a block's weight. Finally, there is a configuration page for blocks where administrators can easily determine if a block should appear *only* on certain pages or if a block should appear everywhere *except* certain pages. For example, if an administrator only wanted the login form to appear on the left-hand column of the home page, that would be configured

FIGURE 4. Block Configuration Page

Block	Enabled	Weight	Placement	Operations
Left sidebar				
Navigation	☑	0	left sidebar	configure
Add Content	☑	0	left sidebar	configure
User login	☑	0	left sidebar	configure
Right sidebar				
Author Information	☑	0	right sidebar	configure

here. Finally, administrators also have the option to hard-code conditions where a block should appear. This last feature provides an almost unlimited set of conditions tests that could be established for the display of content in Drupal.

The themes system and Block Module represent two of Drupal's most powerful features. They grant the power to determine the system content, the formatting, and the conditions under which content will appear in the Drupal publishing system.

THE HEALTH SCIENCES LIBRARIES' IMPLEMENTATION OF DRUPAL

The Selection Process

The implementation of a content management system, while replete with milestones, resists a definitive date of completion. The WCM implementation process is, essentially, ongoing as new features are continually added, new versions implemented, and site configurations are changed over time. With this notion in mind, experience in this process has taken the Health Sciences Libraries Web committee members far beyond their initial understanding of content management. Many aspects of the practice, such as basic content management strategies and approaches, expectations for core functionalities, strategies for identifying and meeting strategic organizational needs, and much more, only revealed themselves in the implementation and management phases of the process. And, while the HSL Web committee has ultimately been pleased with the performance of Drupal as a light-weight CMS (although perhaps not an "official" CMS), many more considerations will find their way into the discovery and selection process of future systems. It is also important to recognize that while the core list of requirements will undoubtedly be more extensive and more formal in future selection processes, the basic philosophy will remain centered on meeting user expectations. With this observation in mind, following is an exploration of the initial selection and discovery process along with discussion of considerations that will make their way into selection of future systems.

If the selection and implementation of a CMS were not already complex, the Health Sciences Libraries added to the difficulty by simultaneously undergoing a major redesign of its Web presence. While the CMS itself would provide new features that could potentially affect design decisions, it is generally not recommended that these two processes coincide, as both require a great deal in the way of time and attention. However, engaging in the redesign process while simultaneously implementing the CMS did result in one important benefit–it rooted the CMS selection strategy in a heavily user-centered design process. That is to say, the Web committee made use of a popular high-level Web development framework, created by a notable information architect, Jesse James Garret, throughout the development and design process. His *Elements of User Experience* emphasizes the need to introduce user-centered strategic thinking early on in the design process, which translated to a focus on user needs in the selection of a CMS as opposed to the perhaps more traditional bias of purely addressing IT systems needs.[6] The primary set of requirements that arose from the initial investigation into staff needs included: WSIWYG editor capability, easy access to update pages to maintain quality, a "forgiving" and usable content contribution interface, enforcement of HTML standards, and revision control. Generally speaking, there was a strong desire among a number of the staff to gain greater access and control over more content on the Web site. Selection criteria such as these acted as a kind of litmus test for the selection process. Content management systems that did not provide these core functionalities were ruled out from the beginning.

As the staff began to investigate content management systems and tools, a basic set of key features arose as points of comparison, both from staff interviews and from observed common features. A ranking matrix was constructed to compare these tools (see Figure 5).

The committee considered a variety of content management systems and tools (primarily tools) and chose Drupal based upon the selection criteria mentioned previously. Such systems included, but were not limited to: Joomla, Xoops, Keystone Digital Library Suite, Macromedia Contribute, and Plone. While there was interest in freely available open source software due to the added benefits of collaboration in open source software development, commercial closed and open source products were also considered. However, the vast majority of commercially available content management systems seemed far beyond the reach of the library budget. Drupal also enjoys a large local following in the Minneapolis-St Paul area, providing the library with opportunities for affordable outside support as well as for informal knowledge sharing with community members. In combining these "intangibles" with the results of the Health Sciences Libraries' internal investigation, Drupal became the clear choice for a library CMS. Since the time of the HSL selection, the IBM Internet Technology Group team has written a

FIGURE 5. Selection Matrix

Matrix Items	Rank (1-5)	Weight (1-5)
1) Editor Interface		5
2) Backend Administration		4
3) Standards Compliant HTML/XHTML templates		4
4) Potential for Outside Support		2
5) Scalability		3
6) Price (affordability)		4
7) Availability for Out-of-Box Add-Ons		3
8) Customizability		4
9) Internal Support Capability		4
10) Security		5

Matrix Key
1-How Usable is the Editor/Contributor Interface?
2-Does the tool provide flexible administration features?
3-Does the system produce valid HTML/XHTML?
4-Can we easily contract others to maintain/upgrade the system?
5-Will it perform at the same level with increased load?
6-Is the system affordable?
7-Are there many available add-ons?
8-How hard is it to add/modify system features & functionality?
9-Does library IT have capacity to support this resource?
10-Is the system sufficiently secure?

series of short articles on implementing Drupal, including a discussion of why they chose to promote Drupal for its ease and robust flexibility in building collaborative Web sites over other content management frameworks such as Mambo <http://www.mamboserver.com/>, Typo3 <http://typo3.com/>, Ruby on Rails <http://www.rubyonrails.org/>, and a variety of blog engines.[7] This sort of endorsement certainly adds to the Health Sciences Libraries' confidence in the power of Drupal to meet the needs of its users.

Future requirements for a content management system will more closely follow the "collection, management, and publishing" features outlined in the preceding discussion. This framework provides a useful means of assessing the abilities of a given content management system, even to evaluate whether or not a given application fully meets the definition of a CMS. More specifically, it stresses the need to examine the capabilities of common content management systems features, such as workflows, content conversion utilities, metadata management features, or templates in order to properly evaluate the effectiveness of a given system. By combining an understanding of these common features with the knowledge of internal user needs, the Health Sciences Libraries staff will have an even better chance at successful CMS implementations in the future.

Drupal and Web 2.0

Web 2.0 may have no definitive definition, but generally it is associated with a more improved, more social Web experience for end users, one that has begun to more fully leverage Javascript and that has begun to allow much greater participation and control for the average Web surfer.[8] Such features have begun to slowly filter into the scholarly community, and grants are beginning to back up research in this area. Casey Bisson of Plymouth University recently won the Mellon Award for Technology Collaboration for his WPopac tool. What makes his project significant is that it ties a traditional library service with a host of new technology approaches that come bundled with the Word Press blog application. Many currently emerging practices on the Web, such as allowing viewers to make comments on site content, resulted from blog-related development. By building a library catalog presence into this environment, Bisson ensures currency with emerging and contemporary Web practices. This same tactic was another deciding factor in the decision of the Health Sciences Libraries to move forward with Drupal after the initial round of investigation had been completed.

Drupal offers a wide variety of "Web 2.0" features either through core features or add-on modules: tagging "folksonomies," comment-enabled content, integration with "social bookmarking" sites (e.g., Del.icio.us), content raking/voting, member profiles for social networking, and more. It is also important to note here that Drupal provides the *option* to utilize these tools. That is, these features may be enabled or disabled, many on a post-by-post basis. The key here is that Drupal possesses the capability as a framework to enable greater user participation and control (comments, user contributed content, user profiles, etc.) within a library environment. Perhaps the best way to stay current with Web trends is to build systems around lightweight, forward-looking content management frameworks such as Drupal.

The Implemenentation

The Health Sciences Libraries' installation of Drupal involved a great deal of work in the areas of Drupal module development and general system configuration. Third-party modules often provided a baseline of functionality that was modified by HSL IT staff to fit the context of the HSL Web site implementation.

Modules–Installed and Built. Perhaps the most labor intensive portion of a Drupal installation pertains to module development where system features must be extended, altered, or added outright. Fortunately, Drupal presents a highly modular system architecture on which to build. In fact, the vast majority of Drupal's power lies within the "module" system, which allows administrators and developers to truly extend Drupal's capabilities. One of the governing principles of Drupal is to keep core system functionality to a minimum, allowing add-on modules to extend features where needed. There are two primary reasons for this approach: (1) it prevents the core system from becoming bloated with too many features, leaving it up to administrators to decide what is really needed in each installation; and (2) by keeping core features to a minimum, core developers can be more agile in regards to upgrading basic system functionality. This latter aspect means Drupal will address emerging trends and meet end-user needs more flexibly, without becoming enslaved by past architectural decisions. The drawback of this approach is that not all modules are maintained with the same level of care, and Drupal administrators may find themselves closely tied to a module that has not made the transition to the latest version of the core Drupal installation. Administrators can hedge against this problem by adopting only those modules with active communities and by offering direct support, where possible, to the ongoing development of these modules.

The Health Sciences Libraries depends upon a variety of popular add-on modules for its Drupal installation. Add-on modules that play a role in operation of the Health Sciences Libraries site include, but are not limited to, such modules as Event, Image, Image Assist, Masquerade, Signup, TinyMCE, and Workspace.

The Event Module is "a simple module to keep track of events and show them to users in various calendar displays."[9] This simple description, however, underplays the significant amount of functionality that the module offers, functionality that became an important part of the Health Sciences Libraries site workshop registration system. All content types in Drupal can be tied to the Event Module calendar, offering many possibilities to create custom content types for events. In the case of the Health Sciences Libraries, a "workshop" content type was constructed and tied to the Event Module. Library workshops, therefore, were able to be registered in a centralized calendar.

The Image Module plays a key role in many Drupal installations. This module allows "users with proper permissions to upload images into drupal."[10] It also automatically generates different sizes of images, for example, "thumbnail" images. The Image Module allows site administrators to configure sizes for these versions, and maximum sizes can be set within the central Drupal upload area.

The Image Assist Module "allows users to upload and insert inline images into posts," and is especially useful where tied to the TinyMCE WYSIWYG ("what you see is what you get") editor.[11] Users can easily upload and insert images directly into pages on which they are working with Image Assist. This module has been invaluable as a mechanism for staff.

The Masquerade Module is focused on helping administrators to manage user settings issues. Administrators can simply navigate to the user account page of a given user and click on a link to "Masquerade" as this user in order to test permissions settings and the like. The role-based permissions structure of Drupal can sometimes make permissions settings complicated. By giving administrators the option of seeing the world as their users, access issues can be checked quickly.

The Signup Module was closely tied to the Event Module in the Health Sciences Libraries implementation, also within the context of the workshop content type. It "allows users to sign up (or register, as in register for a class) for nodes of any type."[12] The Signup Module handles the user registration component of workshops, adding such features as reminder e-mails prior to event times and automatic closing of events based on event date and time. Workshop registrations automatically close in this installation one hour before a given workshop. Finally, users may see classes for which they have registered either by viewing the workshops page while signed into the Drupal system or by viewing their account details, where all registrations appear. Some of these modules, such as the Book Module, will become less important as the HSL moves to a newer version of the system where some of the functionality of these modules has been bundled directly into the core system.

The TinyMCE Module brings the power of the TinyMCE <http://tinymce.moxiecode.com/> editor into Drupal. This "What You See is What You Get" (WYSIWYG) editor provides content contributors with a

Microsoft Word Like authoring tool for Web content in Drupal. Some HSL staff members use this utility for the creation and maintenance of Web pages (see Figure 6). Others simply edit HTML directly. While WYSIWG technology can produce sub-standard HTML and occasionally confusing results for Web amateurs, it does offer a path to managing content for those without the time to master HTML. As a result, the HSL was able to bring more contributors into the management of the Web site, resulting in more buy-in and general success in meeting the original goals of content management at the libraries. Newer versions of the module (Drupal 4.7 and beyond) bundle a much wider set of configuration options as well, including personalized versions of the editor for different user roles.

The Workspace Module provides system users with a "central place to view and manage their content."[13] It became obvious that these features in the core Drupal offerings were both lacking and necessary for the tracking of user contributions. As a result, this module was a welcomed addition to the HSL Drupal installation.

The number of modules that the Health Sciences Libraries make use of far exceeds the brief listing above, but they do represent some of the most important. Of course, other libraries may find other modules more indispensable, depending upon the needs of their own user community. As mentioned, one of the strengths of the system is that it favors configuration and add-ons over a prescriptive, highly inflexible architecture.

Part of this flexibility comes in the ability of developers to simply build their own modules to extend Drupal functionality. As discussed, developers can create new content/node types in Drupal. In doing so, developers are actually creating a new "node module," building on Drupal's module system and allowing them to create highly tailored content authoring interfaces, to add custom features to the content type (e.g., a date selection popup), and to control the style of the output with

FIGURE 6. TinyMCE WYSIWYG Editor

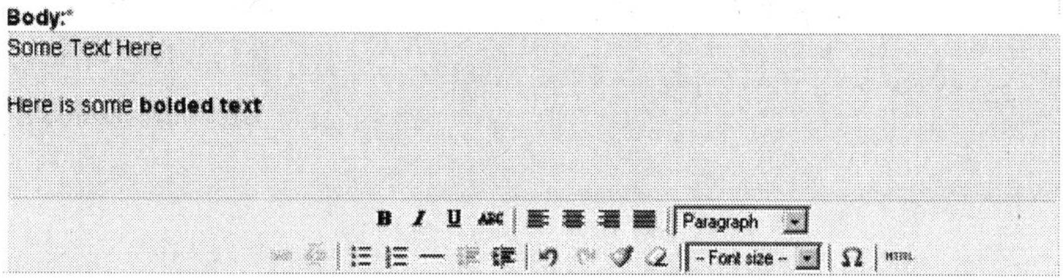

content type-specific templates. This practice may diminish, however, as Drupal has introduced a set of mechanisms for automatically creating new content types without the need to write code: the Content Construction Kit (CCK), which is itself a module. Because of this emerging utility, Drupal developers will be able to produce new content types much more rapidly. Because the CCK module is producing the new content types, the task of system upgrades is easier as only one module must be updated as opposed to one per content type.

Modules are also not limited to creating new content types. Using the Drupal API (application program interface), developers can add an almost limitless range of new features to Drupal. The Drupal API provides a framework for developers such that all coding practices are consistent and organized in a similar fashion from one module to another. Moreover, Drupal provides many basic Web development features, such as role-based user management, output templates, and access control. As a result, developers using Drupal need not create these features each time they want to build a Web application. Rather, they simply tie into a pre-existing framework.

An example of a custom built Drupal module, the HSL Drupal implementation makes use of a module to integrate the Drupal user login framework with a campus-wide authentication authorization system. By building this module HSL users may now simply log into Drupal using the normal campus login process.

HSL Drupal System Configuration. Key aspects of the Health Sciences Libraries' configuration of Drupal involved basic content workflow, user access, and general site configuration.

Effective workflows are likely to track closely to organizational structure. Many medical libraries have adopted team-based work environments, including the Health Sciences Libraries.[14] As a result, it would seem that the flat organizational structure of team-based work environments in libraries mitigates in favor of a relatively shallow hierarchy within the workflow of a given CMS. Pre-publication review should then enforce a minimal level of content review prior to "live" publication of Web pages, particularly where content types are rigidly defined, as these offer a higher level of structure to content contributions via custom input forms. Larger organizations with strict organizational hierarchies will undoubtedly require more stringently hierarchical publication processes.

In the case of the Health Sciences Libraries, the required workflow was relatively uncomplicated. The lack of strict workflow requirements made Drupal a viable CMS candidate for the HSL as Drupal does not possess sophisticated workflow features, although this has begun to change somewhat. Custom content types, such as staff contact pages and workshops pages, are handled by staff members who have been put in charge of these site "sections." The webmaster receives notifications as content is created and can review and modify this content. However, there is not an approval cue for this content; authors are left to self regulate, understanding that some review will take place. It is also important to underscore the fact that with custom content types, the requirements for authors to create their own HTML or otherwise inject styles into the content, is much reduced as custom content types can utilize tailored content intake forms and templates for content output. There is, however, one exception to the lack of an approval cue: library news. Any library content contributor can add news items to the site, but news items will not appear on the library home page until the communications coordinator or webmaster has approved the post. This practice allows these staff members to ensure conformance of the content, both in terms of style and tone.

"Standard" pages are maintained by a variety of staff members, some controlling just a few pages, others monitoring and updating whole sections. Much as with custom content type posts, the webmaster receives e-mail notifications of new and updated content for these pages. There are also staff members who act as "site editors" and have access to all content on the site. This level access allows more highly trained staff members to update broken links or otherwise make time sensitive corrections to the site as needed.

In order to provide staff with a true preview of new page content, the HSL IT staff built a "rollover" module that allows staff to create new versions of a given page on a "staging server" (a Web server that mirrors the content of a live site) where they can see what a given page will look like before moving it to the live server. The module also builds in a notification system for editors as well as a comment log and version tracking system; however, at the time this paper was written, this module was still in active development.

The general site configuration of Drupal comes within the "settings" section of the administration environment. It is here that the system time format is set, for example; however, the vast majority of the decisions that must be made in a Drupal installation actually occur within the administrative settings areas of individual modules, which appear as subsections to the main settings page. A great many configuration options play a role in the Health Sciences Libraries Drupal installation, but it is not possible to address all of these within the context of this discussion. Moreover, there is so much variation in these settings, depending upon the particular needs of a community, that knowledge of the particular choices made at the Health Sciences Libraries may only be marginally useful.

CONCLUSION

Web content management (WCM) comes in seemingly innumerable varieties. The number and scope of considerations in selecting a CMS make the process unapproachable in the extreme for newcomers to the practice. Drupal offers one possible avenue for libraries to begin managing content, particularly where workflow needs are not strict and there is a desire to keep current with trends in Web development. Libraries that would like to explore a Drupal implementation are recommended to consult the implementation guide developed by the IBM Internet Technology Group team at <http://www-128.ibm.com/developerworks/ibm/osource/index.html>.

REFERENCES

1. Yu, H. "Library Web Content Management: Needs and Challenges." In *Content and Workflow Management for Library Web Sites Case Studies*, 1-21. Hershey, PA: Information Science Pub., 2005.

2. Boiko, B. *Content Management Bible*, 2nd ed. Norwod, MA: Books24x7, 2005. Available: <http://library.books24x7.com/book/id_9510/viewer.asp?bookid=9510>. Accessed: November 1, 2006.

3 Suh, P; Addy, D.; Thiemecke, D.; and Ellis, J. *Content Management Systems*. Norwod, MA: Books24x7, 2005. Available: <http://library.books24x7.com/toc.asp?bookid=7514>. Accessed: November 1, 2006.

4. Ragetli, J. "Methods and Tools for Managing Library Web Content." In *Content and Workflow Management for Library Web Sites Case Studies*, 22-49. Hershey, PA: Information Science Pub., 2005.

5. Byron, A. "Revision Moderation | drupal.org." (2006). Available: <http://drupal.org/project/revision_moderation>. Accessed: November 1, 2006.

6. Garrett, J.J. *The Elements of User Experience: User-Centered Design for the Web*. Indianapolis, IN and London: New Riders, 2003.

7. Lewis-Bowen, A.; Evanchik, S.; and Weitzman, L. "Using Open Source Software to Design, Develop, and Deploy a Collaborative Web site, Part 1: Introduction and Overview." (2006). Available: <http://www-128.ibm.com/developerworks/ibm/ library/i-osource1/index.html?ca=drs-#rate>. Accessed: November 1, 2006.

8. Graham, P. "Web 2.0." (2005). Available: <http://www.paulgraham.com/web20.html>. Accessed: November 1, 2006.

9. Killesreiter, G. "Event | drupal.org." (2003). Available: <http://drupal.org/project/event>. Accessed: November 1, 2006.

10. Walker, J. "Image | drupal.org." (2003). Available: <http://drupal.org/project/image>. Accessed: November 1, 2006.

11. Shell, B. "Img_assist | drupal.org." (2004). Available: <http://drupal.org/project/img_assist>. Accessed: November 1, 2006.

12. Wright, D. "Signup | drupal.org." (2005). Available: <http://drupal.org/project/signup>. Accessed: November 1, 2006.

13. VanDyk, J. "Workspace | drupal.org." (2004). Available: <http://drupal.org/project/workspace>. Accessed: November 1, 2006.

14. Martin, E.R. "Team Effectiveness in Academic Medical Libraries: A Multiple Case Study." *Journal of the Medical Library Association* 94, no. 3 (July 2006): 271-8.

doi:10.1300/J115v26S01_08

It's a Wiki Wiki World

Mary Carmen Chimato

SUMMARY. Wikis are an excellent way of sharing information and facilitating teamwork and communication in a library. Wikis enable library staff to collectively contribute, edit, and comment on a Web site and can be implemented in a variety of ways. Internally, a wiki can serve as an institutional knowledgebase or repository. Publicly, a wiki can be an online version of a journal or book club, an interactive resource guide, or a space where certain user groups can share thoughts and suggestions about a common experience or project. This article will provide an introduction to wikis, overview the different software, highlight how one medical library is using its wiki as an organizational knowledgebase, and propose several ways a medical library may enable patrons to utilize wikis. doi:10.1300/J115v26S01_09 *[Article copies available for a fee from The Haworth Document Delivery Service: 1-800-HAWORTH. E-mail address: <docdelivery@haworthpress.com> Website: <http://www.HaworthPress.com> © 2007 by The Haworth Press, Inc. All rights reserved.]*

KEYWORDS. Wikis, social software, medical libraries, communication, teamwork, Library 2.0, staff training

---

Mary Carmen Chimato, MLS, MSIS (mary_chimato@ncsu.edu) is Head of Access and Delivery Services, North Carolina State University's Libraries, 2205 Hillsborough Street, Box 7111, Raleigh, NC 27695-7111. She was formerly Head of Access Services at the Health Sciences Library at Stony Brook University.

[Haworth co-indexing entry note]: "It's a Wiki Wiki World." Chimato, Mary Carmen. Co-published simultaneously in *Medical Reference Services Quarterly* (The Haworth Information Press, an imprint of The Haworth Press, Inc.) Vol. 26, Supp. #1, 2007, pp. 169-190; and: *Medical Librarian 2.0: Use of Web 2.0 Technologies in Reference Services* (ed: M. Sandra Wood) The Haworth Information Press, an imprint of The Haworth Press, Inc., 2007, pp. 169-190. Single or multiple copies of this article are available for a fee from The Haworth Document Delivery Service [1-800-HAWORTH, 9:00 a.m. - 5:00 p.m. (EST). E-mail address: docdelivery@haworthpress.com].

Available online at http://mrsq.haworthpress.com
© 2007 by The Haworth Press, Inc. All rights reserved.
doi:10.1300/J115v26S01_09

THE WIKI WAY

Ward Cunningham defines a wiki as "the simplest online database that could possibly work."[1] While that may be a bit of an oversimplification, it is not too far off the mark. Perhaps a more accurate definition of a wiki would be "a tool that easily facilitates online collaboration and communication." Wikipedia defines a wiki as "a type of software that allows the visitors themselves to easily add, remove, and otherwise edit and change some available content, sometimes without registration"[2] (see Figure 1). The term wiki also refers to the collaborative software that is used to create the site.

Wikis are part of a group of software that promotes social interactions called "social software." As defined by the Wikipedia, "social software enables people to rendezvous, connect or collaborate through computer-mediated communications and to form online communities."[3] The defining features of a wiki include: a space containing pages that can be freely written or edited by anyone, use of WikiWords (an amalgamation of two or more words composed of at least two letters each without intervening white spaces, where the first letter of each component word is capitalized and the remaining letters are in lowercase[4]) to automatically link to a page referred to by that name, and use of a simplified hypertext mark-up language to create and edit pages.[5] By employing WikiWords, the content of a wiki is searchable via keywords.

The Wikipedia is the most well known wiki, with more than 3.8 million articles, over 1.4 million of which are in English. By clicking on the "Edit this Page" tab at the top of the screen, anyone, without having to register and create an account, may add, remove, or change the content

FIGURE 1. The Wikipedia's Definition of Wiki[3]

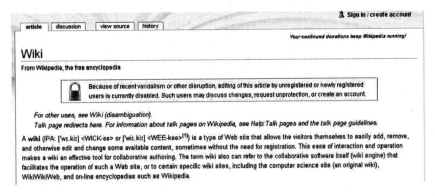

of an article. Content changes can be viewed by clicking the "History" tab, and users may subscribe to alerts that will tell them when a change has been made to a particular page. The "Discussion" tab allows users to discuss and debate content changes and brainstorm ideas for additions or organization of the information in an entry. All of this collaboration is done virtually, in real-time, mostly between strangers, who share a common interest or area of expertise and have the desire to distribute their knowledge.

This collaborative nature of wikis makes them very good tools in organizations that need to share or create a knowledgebase. The real-time updating of content allows quick access to up-to-date information and permits users to distribute this information instantly. Information housed in a wiki may be viewed by the public or, when installed behind a firewall, access can be restricted to only organization or department members.

SO YOU WANNA SURF THE WIKI WAVE?

Libraries can utilize wikis in a number of ways to help organize, promote, and make readily available library resources and services, or to organize library-wide projects or initiatives, as well as aid with interdepartmental communications, policies, and procedures. In order for a library wiki to be successful, the goal, problem, or issue that is to be addressed by its implementation must be clearly defined and understood. For example, if the library's IT coordinator or department would like a place where answers to technical FAQs or a series of troubleshooting steps can be posted to assist staff with technical issues and to help alleviate the amount of time spent fixing small problems, a wiki would be an excellent place to house these documents, while providing a space where staff can discuss the content and give feedback.

Many libraries have chosen to use wikis as organizational knowledge bases. These sites are not available to the public and serve as the holding tank for departmental policies, procedures, organizational goals, project lists, emergency contact information, and many other types of information. Libraries that have chosen to implement semi-public wikis, where patrons can view, but not edit information, have taken their resource guides and made them searchable and easier to navigate by putting them in a wiki. The most well known example of this type of library resource guide wiki is Chad Boeninger's BizWiki at the University of Ohio Libraries <http:// www.library.ohiou.edu/subjects/bizwiki/index.php/Main_Page> (see Figure 2).

FIGURE 2. Main Page of Chad Boeninger's Biz Wiki

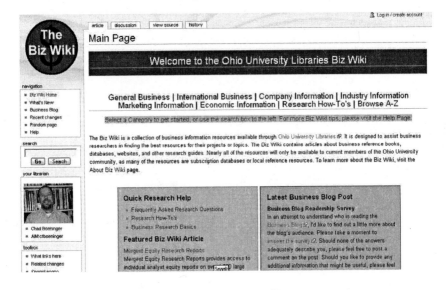

Before creating a wiki, several considerations must be taken into account. As stated above, the problem, goal, or issue must be clearly defined and understood. Once the outcome is clear, the workplace culture and environment must be considered. Who are the users and stakeholders? How comfortable are they with new and emerging technology? Are they tech savvy? Are they willing to invest time in learning a new application? How much training will be needed? Do they believe in the project or will they need to be convinced of its value and usefulness?[6] By discussing and thinking about the answers to these questions now, an organization can save itself many headaches later, and the task of selecting the appropriate software is much easier.

CHOOSING THE RIGHT APPLICATION

Wikis can be created using a variety of different software applications. Currently, there are over 100 different types of wiki software listed on Ward Cunningham's WikiWikiWeb Wiki Engine page <http://c2.com/cgi/wiki?WikiEngines> and on the Wikipedia's List of Wiki Software <http://en.wikipedia.org/wiki/List_of_wiki_software>. When considering the correct software application for your library's wiki, it is important to keep in mind any existing information technology (IT) infrastructure that can be used to support the project.

Is there a server that can house the application or does one need to be purchased? You will need to consider where the wiki will be hosted–in the library by library IT staff or outside the library by a separate company. What computer-scripting language does the wiki employ? The most popular languages are PHP, PERL, ASP, and Python. Is there anyone on staff that understands and can code in these scripting languages? What operating system will be used? Some types of wiki software only run on specific operating systems, so this last point can be very important.[7] The majority of wiki applications are multiplatform and will work provided the basic technical requirements are met; most will inform the user during installation and set-up of any plug-ins or software updates that are missing and need to be installed.

Since a large number of wiki engines are available to users for free, another point that needs to be addressed before choosing an application is whether or not it has all the features and functionality the project requires or that users would like. Two excellent resources to assist in making the software decision are David Mattison's 2003 *Searcher* article[8] and Ward Cunningham's Choosing a Wiki page <http://c2.com/cgi/wiki?ChoosingaWiki>. Mattison's article provides brief overviews of several popular wiki engines, and Cunningham's site provides links to detailed overviews and breakdowns of wiki engines by feature and specifications.

Two final issues to consider are the application's interface and the supporting documentation. The interface and ease of use of the wiki engine will have a direct effect on users' perception and use of the wiki. Wikis employ what is known as wiki markup or wikitext. It is a simplified markup language that indicates various structural and visual conventions.[9] This simplified markup language allows for plain text editing and presents content in a much easier to read format than traditional HTML (see Figure 3).

Most users do not have the time to invest or skills to learn a completely new and unfamiliar online application or programming language. Many newer wiki engines provide What You See Is What You Get (WYSIWYG) text editors that closely resemble the MicroSoft Word interface. These simple editors allow users to create content in the same way they would type a document or send an e-mail message without having to learn a new and unfamiliar set of formatting rules (see Figure 4).

FIGURE 3. Editing Screen Showing the Wiki Markup Language in TWiki

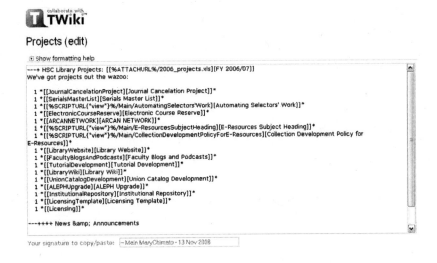

FIGURE 4. Same Page as Figure 3 but Shown Using the WYSIWYG Editor to Create Content

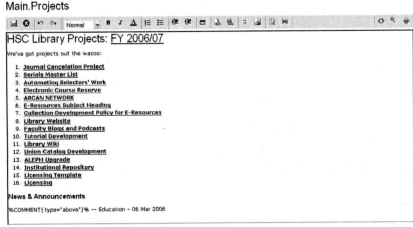

Most wikis also have a Sandbox or Playground feature that allows users to create content without actually publishing it to the wiki. This area is very helpful during wiki training and lets users experiment with the wiki's text formatting, creating numbered and bulleted lists, tables, uploading documents or files, and inserting images. Users can create anything they want on these pages and can change the page's status to "Published" once they have mastered the basics and have created a page they would like to share. In Figure 5, from the Health Sciences Library wiki, the top menu informs users that they are in the Sandbox Web and are free to experiment.

In their 2006 article, Chawner and Lewis point out that a quick, clear picture about the quality of a wiki engine or application can be found by examining the development site and looking over the type of documentation the developers have provided.[7] The user documentation should be easy to understand and supply information regarding the system requirements, installation, upgrade, functionality, and special features of the software. The user's guide should be easy to read and understand by the novice user, readily accessible online and well organized (see Figure 6). Something to keep in mind is that even the best documentation may need to be distilled into simpler instructions for training sessions (see the Appendix).

MAKING A LIBRARY WIKI HAPPEN

Once the goal of the wiki has been identified and the wiki engine has been selected and properly installed, the wiki can be implemented in the library, and staff can then be invited to participate in the project. In order

FIGURE 5. Sandbox Web from the Health Sciences Library Wiki

You are here: TWiki > Sandbox Web > FunWithWikis   r1 - 13 Nov 2006 - 20:15 - MaryChimato

Edit | WYSIWYG | Attach | Printable

This is a test. This is a test of the emergency wiki system.

This is only a test. In the event of an actual emergency:

1. Remain calm.
2. Find the nearest computer.
3. Log in and find out what is going on.
4. ALOHA!

-- MaryChimato - 13 Nov 2006

Edit | WYSIWYG | Attach | Printable | Raw View | Backlinks: Web, All Webs | History: r1 | More topic actions

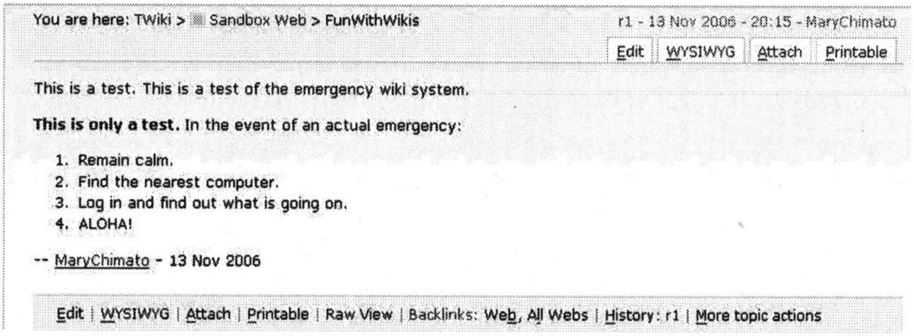

FIGURE 6. The TWiki Web Site Home Page Providing Links to Documentation, FAQs, and Administrative Tools

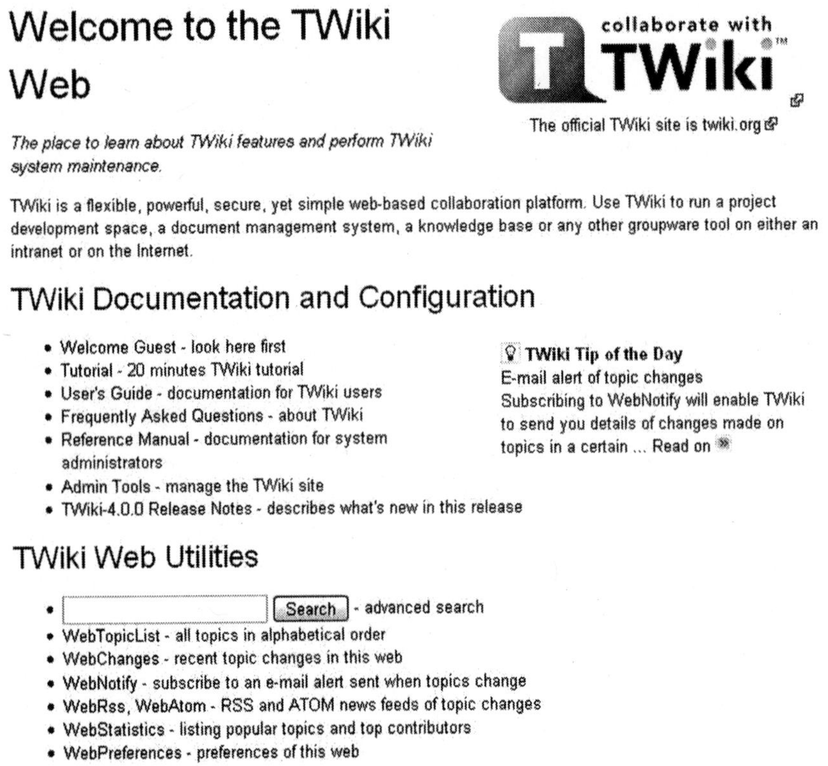

Welcome to the TWiki Web

collaborate with **TWiki**™

The official TWiki site is twiki.org &

The place to learn about TWiki features and perform TWiki system maintenance.

TWiki is a flexible, powerful, secure, yet simple web-based collaboration platform. Use TWiki to run a project development space, a document management system, a knowledge base or any other groupware tool on either an intranet or on the Internet.

TWiki Documentation and Configuration

- Welcome Guest - look here first
- Tutorial - 20 minutes TWiki tutorial
- User's Guide - documentation for TWiki users
- Frequently Asked Questions - about TWiki
- Reference Manual - documentation for system administrators
- Admin Tools - manage the TWiki site
- TWiki-4.0.0 Release Notes - describes what's new in this release

💡 **TWiki Tip of the Day**
E-mail alert of topic changes
Subscribing to WebNotify will enable TWiki to send you details of changes made on topics in a certain ... Read on ➤

TWiki Web Utilities

- [   ] [Search] - advanced search
- WebTopicList - all topics in alphabetical order
- WebChanges - recent topic changes in this web
- WebNotify - subscribe to an e-mail alert sent when topics change
- WebRss, WebAtom - RSS and ATOM news feeds of topic changes
- WebStatistics - listing popular topics and top contributors
- WebPreferences - preferences of this web

for a wiki to be successful, it is vital that the intended participants and users understand the need and importance of the tool. Ideally, all library staff should contribute to the wiki; realistically some will more than others. A great way to ensure participation is to have the project supported from the top down. If the library's administration sees the importance and value of the project and expresses a desire for the wiki to be successful, the staff is more likely to participate. Presenting the project to small groups, such as in department meetings, is a good way to foster excitement and support for the project and will help team members see the value of the wiki as it relates to their department and the library as a whole.

Depending on the purpose of the library's wiki, it may be necessary to "seed" the wiki before staff begins adding content. Seeding the wiki is analogous to creating a table of contents or outline for the wiki. This provides users with examples of the types of materials that are to be included and a schematic for where this information belongs within the wiki.

Staff training and support is essential in order for the wiki to succeed. Training works best in small groups, again possibly at the department level, with clear and concise documentation to support and reiterate what goes on during the hands-on session. The training sessions should be broken down, covering specific topics, becoming progressively more advanced with each session, and should provide users with ample time to play with the functionality and features of the wiki engine. The Sandbox or Playground will provide the space for users to play around in the wiki and familiarize themselves with the type of text formatting the wiki employs. After the initial rounds of staff training have concluded, it is helpful to provide refresher or drop-in sessions where users can ask questions, give feedback, or get help with a specific issue.

WIKI IN ACTION:
THE HEALTH SCIENCES LIBRARY'S WIKI

The Health Sciences Library at Stony Brook University developed a wiki at the beginning of 2006. The library is a medium-sized, academic health sciences library, with 30 full-time staff and between 10 and 12 part-time student employees. The library serves the academic, clinical, and research needs of the University's Medical Center (the School of Medicine and University Hospital) and the four schools comprising the Health Sciences Center (School of Dental Medicine, School of Health Technology and Management, School of Nursing, and School of Social Welfare), as well as the greater university. Looking at the 2006-2007 projects list, it became evident that many library projects were inter-departmental, affecting many different areas of the library, and that communication across departments was essential to the success of most of these projects. Due to the relatively small size of the library and the large number of projects occurring (see Figure 7), communication and skills were very compartmentalized and the availability of written policies and procedures varied by department; therefore, a wiki as a central knowledgebase and information repository seemed like a formidable solution to the communication problem.

The library's Multimedia Applications Group (MAG) reviewed several different wiki engines before selecting TWiki as the application. The library is fortunate to have a large IT department and an outstanding

FIGURE 7. The Project List That Was the Catalyst Behind the Wiki Project

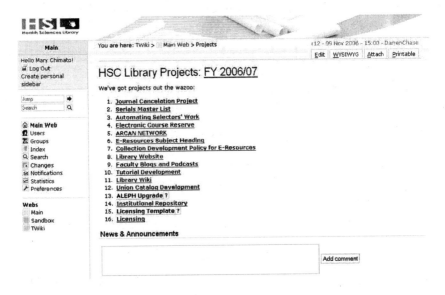

existing infrastructure allowing it to host the wiki internally on a library-owned server and to take advantage of the large variety of skills the library systems department offers. TWiki's features–revision control, ability to upload or download any file as an attachment, online registration of new users, syndication, full-text searching, topic locking, and many others, as well as a wide variety of plug-ins that are available allowing further customization–made it an ideal application for the library.

Since the wiki was a new tool and application for the majority of staff, the applications team decided to seed the wiki to provide a framework for the contents and to illustrate the purpose of the wiki. The applications team created a broad structure for content and provided the foundation for each section of the wiki. Upon completion of wiki training, staff was expected to be responsible for determining and creating the content of their respective sections (see Figures 8 and 9).

The first round of introductory wiki training began in late May 2006 and continued through June. Training was conducted in small groups, by department, and lasted between 45 minutes to an hour depending upon how quickly staff learned basic skills and the number of questions received. It was important for the applications team that the training be an enjoyable experience that staff would discuss with one another and generate word of mouth support for the library wiki. In order to accomplish

FIGURE 8. Part of the Main Page of the Health Sciences Library Wiki Displaying How Staff Seeded the Wiki, Creating an Organizational Structure for Content

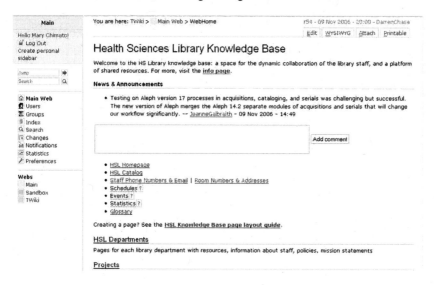

FIGURE 9. The First Phase of Content Created by Members of Resource Management Services

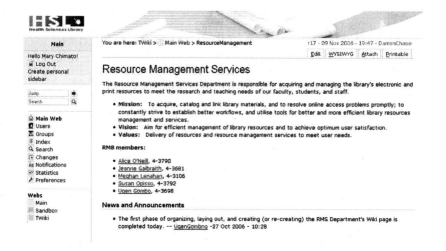

this, training was conducted with a Hawaiian theme. The computer lab was adorned with luau decorations, students received leis when they entered the room, Hawaiian music was played, and the session was short and concise with lots of hands-on experience. Staff members were required to create basic pages in the Sandbox (see Figure 10), utilize lists and insert hyperlinks, and then asked to discuss how their department might utilize the wiki to benefit their workload or the library as a whole.

Wiki training by department paid off in several extremely positive ways. It facilitated communication within each department. Often the training sessions transformed into group brainstorming periods where staff would recommend different applications of the wiki for the department and one another. Open communication often led to a better understanding of the complexities and responsibilities of another staff member's job and day-to-day tasks. In departments lacking written policies, procedures, and workflows, having a place to create and store these documents inspired their creation and in some cases led to revisions and changes to "the way we always did it."

Wiki training also had an effect on inter-departmental communication. Staff members were able to identify specific types of information from other departments that would help them answer patron questions or assist them with an aspect of their job duties. For example, the reference desk often receives calls from patrons inquiring about overdue fines and policies; the librarian on duty can go to the wiki for the information instead of transferring the call to the circulation desk or physically locating someone in circulation to answer the question (see Figure 11).

FIGURE 10. Example of a Staff Page Created in the Sandbox During a Training Session

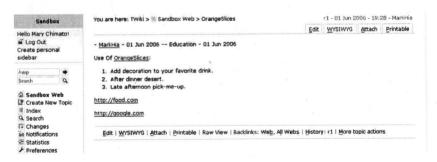

FIGURE 11. Overdue Fines Schedule and Policies Posted on the Library Wiki

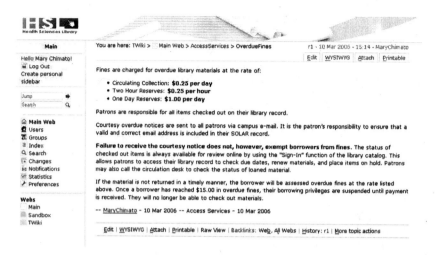

Often members of one department do not know what is happening or what project is being worked on by other departments. Posting the progress of various projects on the wiki was an easy way to keep library staff informed of what was happening throughout the library and helped identify areas that could benefit from cross-department collaboration. Figure 12 shows a progress page created by the Dynamic Applications Team.

After completing and gathering feedback from the initial round of training, it was decided that follow-up training and support needed to be routinely provided to library staff. A simple way to do this was to attend a department's staff meeting on a regular basis to address problems and identify new uses for the wiki. The Multimedia Applications Group introduced "Wiki Wednesdays," where anyone on staff could drop in during a specified time and receive help and additional training. It became very clear that in order for the wiki to be successful, staff needed to feel comfortable in asking for help and know that wiki support was available to them when needed. One of the major selling points of the wiki to the staff was the fact that it cannot be broken; no one, no matter how hard they tried, could irrevocably break the wiki because of the revision control feature. When this fact sunk in, people became more comfortable with playing with features, creating and editing pages.

FIGURE 12. Page Created by Dynamic Applications Team Updating the Scope and Progress of Their Online Tutorial Projects

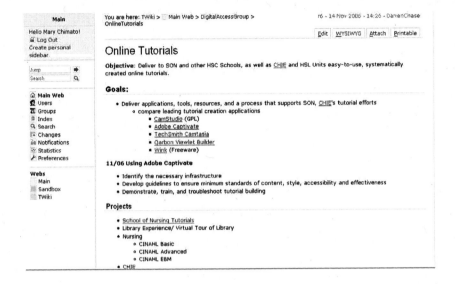

OTHER WAYS TO WIKI

The Health Sciences Library chose to use its wiki to promote communication and collaboration across the organization and to solve an "information overload" problem. An informal survey of the MEDLIB discussion list, conducted in September 2006 to find out how other medical and health sciences libraries were using wikis, yielded surprising results. Many libraries were also using wikis internally as knowledge bases, but almost none were creating or using wikis that were available to the public. Meredith Farkas proposes several public uses for wikis in libraries:[10]

- Subject Guides: Since it can be edited by anyone, patrons can add links to a list of resources and remove dead ones, creating a list of resources that truly represents the interests of the users.
- Annotating the Catalog: Beyond the basic information contained in a MARC record, adding extra content such as a synopsis, cover art, or reviews helps patrons find books that interest them.

- Community wiki: The library's Web site can become the online hub of a community by containing useful community information and links.

Most medical and health sciences libraries are not open to the public and cater to a very specific patron base that at first makes these suggestions seem inapplicable; however, special libraries can take these ideas and customize them to their mission and patrons. Some of the public wikis that the Health Sciences Library is considering implementing in conjunction with a newly designed Web site are:

- *First-Year Medical Student Wiki*: First- and second-year medical students can share experiences and advice about the realities of medical school.
- *Distance Education/Non-Traditional Nursing Student Wiki:* The School of Nursing offers eight online degree programs; this wiki would provide a public space where prospective and current students in these programs can share their online learning experiences and offer advice to others.
- *Medical Book/Journal Club Wiki:* Adding an online dimension to a journal or book club, where those who may not be able to participate face-to-face can now do so virtually.

These wikis would be accessible to the public, allowing them to read, create, and edit content once they have created an account, but library staff would manage the wikis, pruning content if it was inappropriate or outdated.

The library is also looking at new ways to use the internal staff wiki. The librarians actively teach in the library's education program and in several academic programs offered by the different schools of the Health Sciences Center. One of the areas of the wiki currently under development is an educational resources and materials section where librarians post their syllabi, handouts, and educational materials for others to use, revise, and update. There is also discussion of an "Island of Lost Reference Questions" page where questions that come up at the reference desk or in the classroom that require more time and effort than usual can be worked on and added to as staff collectively and collaboratively try to find answers.

WIKI WISELY

A wiki is an exceptional collaborative tool that can be used in a variety of ways within a library. If your library is exploring the possibility of utilizing a wiki, here are several points to keep in mind:

1. **Purpose:** A wiki must have a clearly defined, specific purpose, goal, or problem to solve. It is difficult to promote, support, or participate in the project when it lacks a clear purpose.
2. **Know your environment:** Who are your users? How tech savvy are they? Do they like new technology? What existing IT skills, support, and hardware can be used on this project? Think about the answers to these questions before selecting a wiki engine.
3. **Training, Training, Training:** A wiki is not instantly intuitive to most people. Training is necessary for successful participation in a wiki project. Keep training sessions short and fun, and allow plenty of time for students to play with the application. Regularly schedule follow-up training to reiterate skills and to address problems or concerns.
4. **Have fun:** Think about new and different ways to exploit the collaborative nature of a wiki. Go outside the box and do something radical!

REFERENCES

1. WhatIsWiki. Available: <http://www.wiki.org/wiki.cgi?WhatIsWiki>. Accessed: September 15, 2006.
2. Wikipedia, The Free Encyclopedia. "Wiki." Available: <http://en.wikipedia.org/wiki/Wiki>. Accessed: September 15, 2006.
3. Wikipedia, The Free Encyclopedia. "Social Software." Available: <http://en.wikipedia.org/wiki/Social_software>. Accessed: September 15, 2006.
4. WikiWikiWeb. "Wiki Word." Available: <http://c2.com/cgi/wiki?WikiWord>. Accessed: November 1, 2006.
5. Tonkin, E. "Making the Case for a Wiki." *Airiadne* 42(January 30, 2005). Available: <http://www.ariadne.ac.uk/issue42/tonkin/intro.html>. Accessed: November 9, 2006.
6. Fichter, D. "The Many Forms of E-Collaboration: Blogs, Wikis, Portals, Groupware, Discussion Boards, and Instant Messaging." *Online* 29, no. 4 (2005): 48-50.
7. Chawner, B., and Lewis, P.H.. "WikiWikiWebs: New Ways to Communicate in a Web Environment." *Information Technology and Libraries* 25, no. 1 (2006): 33-43.
8. Mattison, D. "Quickiwiki, Swiki, Twiki, Zwiki, and the Plone Wars: Wiki as PJM and Collaborative Content Tool." *Searcher* 11, no. 4 (2003): 32-48.

9. Wikipedia, The Free Encyclopedia. "Wikitext." Available: <http://en.wikipedia.org/wiki/Wikitext>. Accessed: September 15, 2006.

10. Farkas, M. "Using wikis to Create Online Communities" *WebJunction* (September 1, 2005). Available: <http://webjunction.org/do/DisplayContent?id=11264>. Accessed: November 11, 2006.

doi:10.1300/J115v26S01_09

APPENDIX

WIKI TRAINING MANUAL

HEALTH SCIENCES LIBRARY WIKI STAFF TRAINING

MAY/JUNE 2006

Table of Contents:

What is a Wiki?

More than simply Hawaiian for "quick," a wiki is a very powerful collaborative tool!

The term wiki is the shortened form of *wiki wiki* (weekie weekie) which is from the native language of Hawaii where it is commonly used as an adjective to denote something "quick" or "fast". In English it is an adverb meaning to do something "quickly" or "fast".

In web terms, a wiki is a type of website that allows users to easily add, remove, or otherwise edit all content very quickly and easily. This ease of interaction and operation makes a wiki an effective tool for collaborative writing. The term **wiki** can also refer to the collaborative software that facilitates the operation of such a website.

In essence, a wiki is a simplification of the process of creating HTML pages combined with a system that records each individual change that occurs over time, *so that at any time, a page can be reverted to any of its previous states.* A wiki system may also include various tools, designed to provide users with an easy way to monitor the constantly changing state of the wiki as well as a place to discuss wiki content. A wiki enables documents to be written collectively in a very simple markup language using a web browser. A single page in a wiki is referred to as a "wiki page," whilst the entire body of pages, which are usually highly interconnected via hyperlinks, is "the wiki"; in effect, a wiki is a very simple, easy-to-use user-maintained database for searching information. The HS Library uses Twiki software to maintain our wiki. Twiki is a type of open source software that is mainly used in commercial environments, often on corporate intranets. Some companies who use Twiki: Disney, British Telecom, SAP and Motorola.

Twiki builds on the original wiki concept and adds a number of features that make it very useful. Twiki pages are fully revision controlled; a record of every change to every page is kept and the look and feel is configurable through the use of templates and plugins.

Basic Twiki can be used as a whiteboard, document repository, collaborative authoring environment, chat, or a notebook/scrapbook. Using Twiki with extensions can produce a content management system for websites, a presentation development tool, a blog, a database, a project management system or a tracking tool. The possibilities are limited to your imagination!

Setting up Your Account and Logging In

To create and edit pages on our Twiki site, you must have a registered user name and password. To do this, go to the following webpage: <*web address where the wiki is hosted*> and complete the registration form.

Registration

To edit pages on this TWikiSite, you must have a registered user name and password.

- 🔲 **Note:** Registered users can ChangePasswords and ResetPasswords.

To register as a new user, simply fill out this form:

Important: the information provided in this form will be stored in a database on the TWiki server. This database is accessible to anyone who can access the server through the web (though passwords will be encrypted, and e-mail addresses will be obfusticated to help prevent spamming). Your country, or the country where the server is hosted, may have Data Protection laws governing the maintenance of such databases. If you are in doubt, you should contact webmaster@example.com for details of the Data Protection Policy of this TWiki server before registering.

Field	Input	
First Name:		**
Last Name:		**
(identifies you to others) WikiName:		**
E-mail address:		**
Your password:		**
Retype password:		**
Organisation name:		
Organisation URL:		
Country:	Select... ⌄	**
Comments: (optional)		

Mashing Up the Internet

Michelle A. Kraft

SUMMARY. Mashups are blended applications combining two or more existing programs to produce a third program offering a unique view and distribution of information or enhancement of services. Currently the most popular mashups today use mapping programs to illustrate and present data. With the growth of software, tools, and common programming languages and platforms, mashups have begun to explode on to the Internet. Their creation and utilization within medical research and libraries is discussed along with concerns regarding data and security. doi:10.1300/J115v26S01_10 *[Article copies available for a fee from The Haworth Document Delivery Service: 1-800-HAWORTH. E-mail address: <docdelivery@haworth press.com> Website: <http://www.HaworthPress.com> © 2007 by The Haworth Press, Inc. All rights reserved.]*

KEYWORDS. Mashups, API, Web 2.0, Internet applications

Michelle A. Kraft, MLS, AHIP (mkraft@cchseast.org) is Medical Librarian, South Pointe Medical Library, 20000 Harvard Road, Warrensville Heights, OH 44122. Michelle Kraft is the author of The Krafty Librarian blog <http://www.kraftylibrarian. blogspot.com/>.

[Haworth co-indexing entry note]: "Mashing Up the Internet." Kraft, Michelle A. Co-published simultaneously in *Medical Reference Services Quarterly* (The Haworth Information Press, an imprint of The Haworth Press, Inc.) Vol. 26, Supp. #1, 2007, pp. 191-207; and: *Medical Librarian 2.0: Use of Web 2.0 Technologies in Reference Services* (ed: M. Sandra Wood) The Haworth Information Press, an imprint of The Haworth Press, Inc., 2007, pp. 191-207. Single or multiple copies of this article are available for a fee from The Haworth Document Delivery Service [1-800-HAWORTH, 9:00 a.m. - 5:00 p.m. (EST). E-mail address: docdelivery@haworthpress.com].

INTRODUCTION

The rise in recent years of social and collaborative software such as wikis, blogs, podcasts, RSS, and folksonomies are commonly bundled as Web 2.0 technology. Medical and library professionals increasingly utilize these technological tools as a means for educational and collaborative endeavors. This collaboration has led to a revolution of innovation where some professional programmers and computer technical savvy individuals delve into the programming of various open source applications and modify them to serve their needs, often combining multiple Web applications and tools resulting in an entirely new program known as a mashup. Over the course of a few short years, mashups have managed to have a profound and dynamic impact on how information and data is displayed, utilized, and shared. Mashups are emerging within the medical and scientific community as well as the library community. This paper will examine the background of mashups and some of their current and potential uses within the medical, scientific, and library information community.

WHAT IS A MASHUP?

The term mashup is derived from the music community where musicians would sample and remix multiple song tracks, vocals, and sounds to create a new song. A Web mashup is a Web site or application that combines data from at least two or more sources creating a seamless separate application or service unique to contributing components. The mashup's contributing data sources can originate from open source applications, from application programming interfaces (APIs) provided by companies such as Google or Yahoo, or from proprietary data from private entities. Programmers have traditionally tried to combine various applications creating a new program; however, it is now easier to do because many of today's mashups use common languages such as JavaScript and XML and frameworks such as AJAX. According to Nathan Lake,

> Mashups have only recently gained a foothold online because their arrival, for the most part, depended on Web site developers' ability to fully utilize these technologies associated with Web 2.0 and take advantage of the free API software and database for public use. By using free API tools developers have been able to interface

one program with another (or more) in order to combine their purposes and create a new way to look at information.[1]

Growth of Mashups

According to the Web site ProgrammableWeb.com <http://program mableweb.com>, approximately 2.90 mashups are created each day.[2] The ChicagoCrime.org site <http://www.chicagocrime.org> is often thought of as one of the first mashups. This site combines data from the Chicago Police Department's Citizen ICAM Web site and Google Maps. ChicagoCrime.org, developed by Adrian Holovaty, allows users to search specific locations by zip code and wards for specific types of crime and dates. Residents cannot only view what types of crimes occurred in their neighborhood and when, but they also can use the route feature to create driving routes specifically avoiding high crime areas. Mapping mashups like ChicagoCrime.org appear to be the more popular type of mashups created. ProgrammableWeb, a site that not only tracks but also allows users to search for the latest mashups and available APIs, reports that 45% of mashups are tagged as mapping mashups (see Figure 1).[3]

The number of mashups created will continue to grow as more and more companies make their APIs publicly available to programmers. Companies such as Google, Yahoo, Amazon.com, and eBay make these APIs available as another method to promote their site. For example, SecretPrices.com <http://www.secretprices.com/> is a Web site that allows users to price comparison shop, search for online coupons, and look at product reviews all using data from Amazon.com, Shopping.

FIGURE 1. Top Mashup Tags

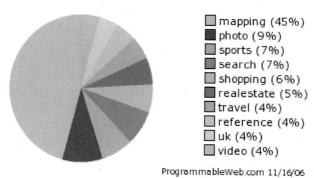

☐ mapping (45%)
■ photo (9%)
☐ sports (7%)
■ search (7%)
☐ shopping (6%)
■ realestate (5%)
☐ travel (4%)
☐ reference (4%)
☐ uk (4%)
☐ video (4%)

ProgrammableWeb.com 11/16/06

com, and Epinions.com. Users are not the only ones who benefit from these new blended Web sites. Lake states that companies like these promote their APIs to "improve sales of their retail products and services."[1] Therefore, it is neither accidental nor completely altruistic that some of the largest and most popular Internet companies are providing and promoting their available APIs.

CAN ANYONE CREATE A MASHUP?

Building a mashup is not as easy as creating a blog or wiki using software packages. It requires programming skills and is still thought to be more of a "programmer's affair" according to ProgrammableWeb.[4] Yet, with the multiple APIs available, common programming languages, and frameworks, it is a lot easier and quicker to create dynamic, lightweight applications that serve a specific need. Many mashups use one or many of the following programming languages: JavaScript, XML, PHP, DHTML, and the AJAX framework. If programming knowledge is not an obstacle, the ProgrammableWeb lists the following steps to create a mashup: pick a subject and evaluate needed coding skills, find data sources, sign up for APIs, and coding.[4]

Mashup Subject and Coding Skills

As Darlene Fichter says, "Content is critical in deciding what mashup to create. What would your users find interesting, engaging, and helpful."[5] There must be an underlying unmet need that the mashup will help solve. Whether it is a mashup that plots all of the McDonald Playlands on Google Maps to wear out the tots on a long family car trip or it is a mashup similar to one used by Pratt & Whitney that enables employees to access and track orders, repairs, and the service history of aircraft engine parts, the end result must serve a defined need.[6] The need defines the type of mashup to be created, which in turn determines APIs and the type of tools necessary to create the program, such as maps, news, and auctions.

In addition to determining the service and type of mashup created, the developer's coding skills should be considered. Even though APIs make coding simpler and are usually "language-agnostic," there are some APIs such as Flickr that use specific programming languages.[4] Simple is sometimes better when first creating a mashup. The beauty of blended applications such as mashups is that they are considered to be lightweight applications and can easily serve a temporary need as well. Developers looking for ideas can browse through ProgrammableWeb's list of over 1,200 mashup applications and brief descriptive information on each application as well as the APIs used.

Data Sources

It all comes down to data. According to ProgrammableWeb, data drives the type of APIs that will be needed to construct the mashup. There are over 300 APIs listed on ProgrammableWeb for developers to browse through, allowing them to view information about each API, such as protocols, security, support, licensing, functionality, as well as a list of other mashup applications using that specific API. The information for each listed API varies; some such as eBay contain detailed information, while FedEx has little.[4] For example, ChicagoCrime.org relies upon data from Google Maps and the Chicago Police Department's Citizen ICAM Web site. One key data question to answer is whether there are APIs already in existence and available for use, such as the case with Google or whether a programmer will be responsible for inputting the data. Not all data is available in public databases as was the case with the data on avian-flu outbreaks within the flu mashup created by Declan Butler for *Nature*. Butler describes his difficulties obtaining the outbreak data in his blog post, "Avian flu maps in Google Earth." Much of the data was compiled by Butler himself.

No single database, or precise spatial data on cases could be obtained from WHO because, it says this would require the lengthy process of it requesting permission to provide it from each affected country. I found locations for many cases in WHO bulletins, although these case data, which come from governments, often themselves provide no detail of even where the case came from, let alone their clinical or epidemiological characteristics–locations were found here by cross-checking cases described in WHO updates with case descriptions in the literature, using dates, sex, and age to identify distinct cases.[7]

Even if the data exists in a database, issues of ownership, security, and reliability can be major factors. Whether the mashup is created for public use or is intended for use behind a company firewall, the issue of ownership must be addressed. While there are many APIs available on the Internet, each have their own licensing and usage requirements. For example, Dun and Bradstreet Business Verification API requires a commercial license and usage fees, while the United States Postal Service API does not require a license agreement and is free.[2] Other companies' license agreements vary according to whether it is a commercial or non-commercial endeavor, such as Google, whose "service may be used only for services that are generally accessible to consumers without charge."[8]

Galen Gruman compares data security and privacy to Pandora's box, because mashups are relatively easy to create compared to some traditional programs and many rely on JavaScript, which is prone to security issues.[6] There have yet to be established clear rules or standards on data and it appears that it is often left up to the original data provider. Data security was a central theme at the Computer-Human Interaction conference in Montreal, Canada, where Hart Rossman, chief security technologist for Science Applications International of Vienna, Virginia, warned that because mashup developers do not own the data, many are just not looking at data integrity, security, and privacy. Data could actually be coming from a hacker's spoof site feeding false data into the application.[9] Libraries hold patron privacy appropriately sacred, so it is a special concern that many APIs have little or no rules as to what developers can do with the data, potentially exposing people's personal information. In the article, "Data Mining 101: Finding Subversives with Amazon Wishlists," Tom Owad demonstrates how easily a mashup can be created using available data within Amazon.com and Google Maps to invade people's privacy. He used Amazon.com's wishlists, which often contain a person's full name, city, and state, to find his or her full address and phone number from Yahoo People Search. Owad described how this data could be easily combined with Google Maps information to provide a satellite image of the person's residence. He then used this information to create a map of people who liked to read "subversive" or "dangerous" literature. Owad spent no money on this project; all that was needed was 30 hours of his time.

All the tools used in this project are standard and free. The services, likewise, are all free. The technical skills required to implement this project are well within the abilities of anybody who has done any programming. The network connection used to download these files was a standard home DSL connection. The computer that processed the data was a 1.5 GHz PowerBook G4. The operating system is Mac OS X 10.4, though everything could have been done just as easily with Linux (and probably with Windows).[10]

Mashup applications are only as strong as their weakest link; often, unreliable or faulty data is that weak link. There are risks with merging integral business applications with third-party data. Eric Lundquist asks the question,

> If your mashed-up sales and marketing system suddenly conks out, who should you blame? Is it Salesforce.com's recently balky hosted customer relationship management offering? Or the companies that have built applications tied in to the Salesforce API? Or maybe it is simply your own Web connection sputtering along?[11]

Depending on what task the mashup is intending on serving, it may behoove companies and institutions to enter into formal license agreements with data providers ensuring integrity and reliability of the information.

API Sign Up and Coding

While there are many APIs available for programmers to use, most require the programmer to sign up or create a user account. For most API providers, it is a quick but necessary process, and the developer can then begin creating and coding the mashup. ProgrammableWeb recommends using the API-specific tutorials. Many of the API providers have detailed and well-written tutorials, guides, and information for using their specific APIs.[2] Google Maps provides extensive documentation including an API upgrade guide from version 1 to version 2, introductions, examples, troubleshooting, and even a discussion group.[8] Other mashup tutorials available for programmers can be helpful as well, such as: "How To Build a Maps Mash-up" by Dan Theurer,[12] and "Screencast: Drupal Mashup Machine" by Zack Rosen.[13] Talis, a provider of library management information systems in the United Kingdom, which sponsored the Mashing Up the Library Competition, also provides links to various APIs, tools, and advice, including APIs for the Talis Platform.

MASHUPS IN MEDICINE AND LIBRARIES

Even though mashups are still relatively new tools to enter the Web 2.0 arena, their dynamic nature and rapid creation have made them an interesting resource tool in the medical and science fields as well as the library field. Mashups offer an opportunity for scientists to combine different bits of information into one application, presenting an overall picture illustrating the possible interactions and dynamics of scientific and medical information. Mashups offer librarians the possibility of displaying and searching for data quicker and expanding services. As Darlene Fichter says, mashups are part of the "customer created content" revolution.[14]

Mashups in Science and Medicine

The ability to create flexible, inexpensive, lightweight applications that can track, collect, and display multiple data sets and information offers enormous possibilities for the scientific and medical community. In his article, "Mashups Mix Data into Global Service," Butler[15] illustrates how researchers can use data to track epidemics, disease patterns, and progression, as he did with his Avian-Flu mashup. Butler's opinion is that this is the first online map offering a visualization of the more than 1,800 avian flu outbreaks in birds that have been reported over the past two years while also providing a visual geographical overview of confirmed human cases of H5N1 influenza infection.[7] Using this information, scientists and medical professionals can better understand the spread of the H5N1 virus in birds and compare it with information on human cases.

HEALTHmap: Global disease alert mapping system is another mapping mashup (see Figure 2). Created by Clark Freifeld and John Brownstein, it combines various data sources mapping disease outbreak information. As the creators say, "HEALTHmap provides a jumping-off Point for real-time information on emerging infectious disease and has particular interest for public health officials and international travelers."[16]

Other medical mapping mashups, such as Berkeley-area Doctors, and Vimo, are targeted at the consumer rather than scientists and researchers. Both programs help the user locate doctors or hospitals and display their locations on either Yahoo or Google Maps. Berkeley-area Doctors only looks specifically for doctors in the Berkeley, California region, and searchers must register using their Aetna policy or subscriber social security number to find more information about the health care provider. Vimo, originally known as Healthia, considers itself an "integrated comparison-shopping portal for healthcare products and services."[17] Businesses and consumers can research, rate, purchase health insurance plans, health savings accounts, and find doctors throughout the United States. Vimo combines private and public data sources enabling searchers to find physicians and compare hospital prices for medical procedures. Additionally, Vimo users can read and post reviews

FIGURE 2. HEALTHmap <http://www.healthmap.org>

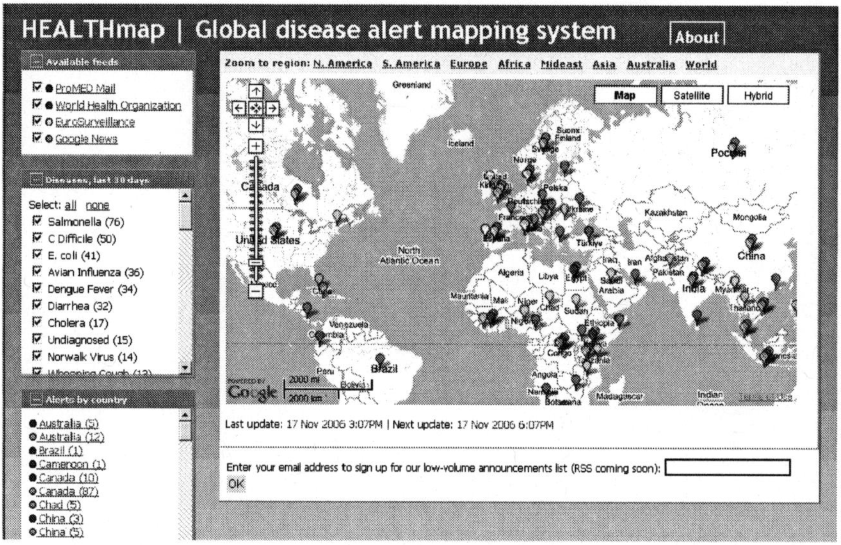

about any of the services or products available.[17] While Vimo is interesting, it still appears to have some flaws. A search for hospital costs for childbirth in the Cleveland, Ohio area yielded no hospitals treating childbirth despite the existence of the three major medical facilities and numerous community hospitals which were later found on Vimo doing an ordinary location search. Again the issue of data becomes critical to the overall mashup product. One program requires users to register using health care policy information with no clear policy regarding its collection, distribution, or privacy, while the other program appears to have missing data regarding medical procedures and hospitals.

Data for some of these mashups can be difficult to obtain due to the sheer amount of information and the fact that it might be located in multiple public and private databases that often do not communicate with each other. However, GenBank, the NCBI genetic sequence database, and UniProt, a central repository of protein sequence and function, have begun to make their data more readily available, allowing those interested in creating genetic mashups more opportunities. The mashup iSpecies by Roderick Page uses data from GenBank. Still in the experimental stages, Page describes iSpecies as "a test of E O Wilson's idea of a web page for each species."[18] Despite this, it shows the possibilities of what can be accomplished combining multiple databases. iSpecies retrieves genomic sequencing information from NCBI, images from Yahoo Images, and articles from Google Scholar. It almost appears that iSpecies resembles an early version of federated searching for researchers primarily interested in genetic sequencing. Users can search for the common name of an animal or the scientific name; however, results vary according to which name is searched, and not all of the articles retrieved will be relevant to the search term. For example, a search for "elephant" yielded genetic information as well as pictures about the animal, and the documents from Google Scholar retrieved topics varying from birth defects to elephant seals. A search for "Elephas maximus," Asiatic elephant, yielded more precise document results. While most of the literature used animals as search examples, iSpecies could be especially helpful to those researching microorganisms. A search for the commonly found Escherichia coli bacteria produced a link to genetic information from NCBI, color images, and articles that Google Scholar retrieved from PubMed. While, this mashup is clearly in the beginning stages, it represents the type of information that mashups can distribute and share to the medical and scientific community to better promote collaboration and research.

Library Mashups

It appears that mashups made a grand entrance into the library community with the 2006 Talis Mashing Up the Library Competition. The competition sought programs that took modern approaches to providing library services, data, and applications online. Paul Miller of Talis says, "The library system can be considered as an interlocking set of functional components rather than a monolithic black box. A new approach can also be taken how information from and about libraries is 'owned' by and exposed to others."[19] The black box Miller refers to is the notion that information is trapped inside a library's catalog, databases, and other systems, and patrons are unable to utilize it with other online non-library tools such as, but not limited to, Amazon.com, MySpace, Flickr, del.icio.us, and Google. While libraries have been making some progress to expand access to their information and services, mashups offer another approach to enhance online information services to patrons. Eighteen entries were submitted to the competition from academic, public, and commercial libraries representing the United States, Canada, Denmark, and the United Kingdom. There were no submissions from medical libraries.

The type of mashups varied from simple enhancements of library functions, to complex collaborative endeavors in online virtual worlds such as Second Life.

The winning mashup entry was awarded to John Blyberg of Ann Arbor District Library in Ann Arbor, Michigan. His creation, the Go-Go-Google-Gadget, puts Ann Arbor District Library feeds into Google's home page for patrons. Google's personalized home page allows users to create gadgets or panels listing information such headlines, weather, etc. Blyberg's gadget takes library information and displays it on the personalized Google home page. Four gadgets are available: hottest library items, newest library material, currently checked-out items, and requested material.[20] Library patrons are no longer forced to go to the library catalog to locate something as simple as their circulation record. Miller describes Blyberg's mashup gadget as "an excellent example of taking information previously locked inside the library catalogue and making it available in other contexts where they may spend more time than they do in their catalogue."[19] This library mashup shifts library services once available only from the library Web site to a popular Web search page that patrons most likely use more often.

Umlaut, by Ross Singer, the winner of The Second OCLC Research Software Contest, is an OpenURL Link Resolver "intended to improve access to library collections by contextualizing citations and available holdings more accurately for a given user."[21] Locating full-text articles can be a time consuming and difficult process. OpenURL Link Resolver programs help library patrons in their full-text searches, but Umlaut goes beyond most standard OpenURL Link Resolver programs. Umlaut analyzes the citation using standard identifiers (currently just DOIs and PMIDs), verifies it through authority sources such as CrossRef and PubMed, and collects the citation's metadata. Umlaut takes the metadata and submits requests to the library link resolver, catalog, and the state union catalog. If there is an ISBN, it will search Amazon.com, Google, and Yahoo. The patron sees brief citation information in the main screen, and quick links on the right-hand side provide more in-depth information upon the patron request. The citation's metadata indicates whether the citation is a book, article, conference proceeding, or a preprint. The "description" link is displayed for book and journal article citations. In the case of a journal article, the PubMed abstract is displayed as the description, and Amazon.com for books. The link "web search results" displays search results for the citation from Yahoo. A demo of how Umlaut works with book citations can be found at <http://umlaut.library.gatech.edu/go/522>, and journal article citations at <http://umlaut.library.gatech.edu/go/523> (see Figure 3). Umlaut is an Open Source application, meaning other enterprising libraries can download it and adjust it for their needs and users.

Many other library mashups, such as Book Burro and Amazon2OU, are centered on finding books. Both of these mashups are plugins for Firefox that, once installed, provide "pivot browsing" to patrons looking for books.[22] While the mechanics are slightly different with these two mashups, they both direct a patron who is looking for a book, or who is simply on a Web page containing a book, to the listing prices from online bookstores and sellers, as well as to information about whether that book is owned by the patron's library. The mashup "pivots" the patron back to the library's catalog and services (see Figures 4 and 5).

FIGURE 3. Umlaut Demo <http://umlaut.library.gatech.edu/go/523>

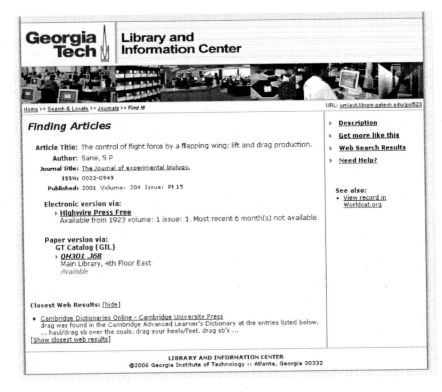

Georgia Tech | Library and Information Center

Home >> Search & Locate >> Journals >> *Find It!*   URL: umlaut.library.gatech.edu/go/523

Finding Articles

Article Title: The control of flight force by a flapping wing: lift and drag production.
Author: Sane, S P
Journal Title: The Journal of experimental biology.
ISSN: 0022-0949
Published: 2001 Volume: 204 Issue: Pt 15

Electronic version via:
  ▶ Highwire Press Free
  Available from 1923 volume: 1 issue: 1. Most recent 6 month(s) not available.

Paper version via:
  GT Catalog (GIL)
  ▶ QH301 .J68
  Main Library, 4th Floor East
  Available

Closest Web Results: [hide]

• Cambridge Dictionaries Online - Cambridge University Press
  drag was found in the Cambridge Advanced Learner's Dictionary at the entries listed below.
  ... haul/drag sb over the coals. drag your heels/feet. drag sb's ...
  [Show closest web results]

▶ **Description**
▶ **Get more like this**
▶ **Web Search Results**
▶ **Need Help?**

See also:
• View record in Worldcat.org

LIBRARY AND INFORMATION CENTER
©2006 Georgia Institute of Technology ¦¦ Atlanta, Georgia 30332

FIGURE 4. Book Burro Firefox Plugin

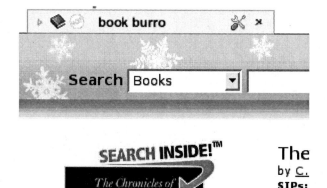

FIGURE 5. Book Burro Firefox Plugin with Price and Library Information

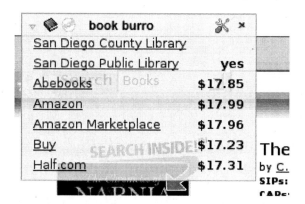

PubMed Mashups

Mashups using NCBI Entrez API and other medical databases and services offer great opportunities to medical libraries as well as medical and scientific professionals. Currently, there are already PubMed knowledge-based search engines offering users their own unique method of searching the PubMed database; however, not all are exactly considered mashups in the strictest sense of the term. PubWindows

<http://www.neurotransmitter.net/pubmed_browser.php?topheight=40>
allows searchers to look for citations within PubMed using a modified
version of the National Library of Medicine's MeSH Database. The top
window displays the altered PubMed browser in which the user types
the desired MeSH term. The bottom window displays check boxes from
which the searcher can enable certain features to appear, such as show
abstracts, show export formats, view SFX demo links, view University
of Illinois at Urbana-Champaign SFX links, and View Northwestern
University SFX links. The information in the bottom window disap-
pears as soon as the user conducts a search and the citations fill the bottom window. The information displayed is structured according to what
features the user enabled from the check boxes at the beginning of the
search. Therefore, if the user activated abstracts, export formats, and
SFX links, those are displayed just below the citation information. One
might argue that the PubMed database already has these display features
while offering a better search interface. However, PubWindows integrates
three other PubMed text mining tools: Chilibot, XplorMed, and BioIE,
allowing the user to search these tools as well. All three of these tools
are word association programs. For example, Chilibot is designed for

> rapidly identifying relationships between genes, proteins, or any
> keywords that the user might be interested. In contrast to the
> PubMed interface where results are organized based on articles,
> Chilibot directly presents the key information user is seeking, i.e.,
> sentences containing both of the terms. These sentences are orga-
> nized into different relationship types based on linguistic analysis
> of the text.[23]

Chilibot can batch process a large number of terms, and those relationships are then summarized as a graph, with links to sentences describing
the relationships, as well as the terms themselves. Using the citation information within the PubMed database, Chilibot, XplorMed, and BioIE
perform an entirely different type of search. As mashups become more
mainstream, and programmers as well as users search for more ways to
synthesize information, look for more mashup applications using PubMed.

THE FUTURE OF MASHUPS IN MEDICINE AND LIBRARIES

Mashups, blended applications, plugins, etc. allow programmers to
create relatively simple and adaptable programs to meet a specific need.
As Open Source programs continue to grow and companies such as

Google, Yahoo, and Amazon.com offer access to their APIs, people will develop new and interesting programs based on their immediate needs. Think of a mashup that allows somebody to conduct a PubMed search displaying not only the citations but also news articles based on those citations, links to cited articles, and other useful information. Perhaps a mashup mapping the location of current clinical trials while including research articles from the principle investigators as well as other research articles on similar studies is just around the corner. Look for more libraries to create mashups enabling patrons to utilize library services not only outside of the library building but also away from the library home page, bringing services and information on demand to patrons where they use it most. It would not at all be inconceivable for other library management systems vendors to follow Talis and release certain APIs to licensed and approved libraries for the purpose of augmenting and further customizing their systems. Perhaps APIs will become another item to be added to vendor contracts, negotiations, and licensing. Competitions like those from Talis and OCLC have only begun to scratch the surface as to what creative programming library professionals can accomplish, and point to what is possible in the future.

CONCLUSION

Mashups are another example of new Web 2.0 technologies and applications shaping the ways medical and library professionals find and provide information. They extend and transform otherwise traditional services. Now, more than ever, information services are expected to be created on demand and to be personalized. The underlying data is the backbone behind these mashup applications; it is what enables these programs to be as multifaceted and relevant as they are. Much of the medical and library communities' data is locked behind private sources or otherwise inaccessible. The private database vendors may be loath to allow data to be accessible or to release their APIs enabling a mashup to be created with another competitor's information. Expect mashups to continue growing at a phenomenal rate using free or available APIs found within public databases, such as ones like GenBank, and from private companies who have much to gain from public use and exposure, such as Google, Yahoo, and Amazon.com. Essentially, the mashup programs formed from these APIs will begin to pave the way for more mashups from within companies and set the stage for the licensing, copyright, ownership, and security issues that many private companies will demand. Only when those issues are resolved will more and more private companies and database vendors be more willing to license, most likely for a fee, their APIs and data to mashup applications. However, that time will come and librarians, medical researchers, and the public will all benefit from these programs.

REFERENCES

1. Lake, Nathan. "Mashups: Melting Pots of Search Tools." *Smart Computing in Plain English* 17(September 2006): 47-9.
2. ProgrammableWeb. Available: <http://www.programmableweb.com>. Accessed: November 22, 2006.
3. ProgrammableWeb. "Mashup Dashboard." Available: <http://www.programmableweb.com/mashups>. Accessed: November 22, 2006.
4. ProgrammableWeb. "How to Make Your Own Web Mashup." Available: <http://www.programmableweb.com/howto>. Accessed: November 22, 2006.
5. Fichter, Darlene. "Doing the Monster Mashup." *Online* 30, no. 4 (July/August 2006): 48-50.
6. Gruman, Galen. "Enterprise Mashups." *InfoWorld* 28, no. 31 (July 31, 2006): 19-23.
7. Butler, Declan. "Avian Flu Maps in Google Earth." Declan Butler, reporter blog. Available: <http://declanbutler.info/blog/?p=16>. Accessed: November 22, 2006.
8. "Google Maps API Terms of Use." Google Maps. Available: <http://www.google.com/apis/maps/terms.html>. Accessed: November 22, 2006.
9. Marks, Paul. "'Mashup' Websites are a Dream Come True for Hackers." *New Scientist* 190, no. 2551 (May 13, 2006): 28-9.
10. Owad, Tom. "Data Mining 101: Finding Subversives with Amazon Wishlists." Applefritter. Available: <http://www.applefritter.com/bannedbooks>. Accessed: November 22, 2006.
11. Lundquist, Eric. "Don't Let Mashups Smash Up." *eWeek* 23, no. 6 (February 6, 2006): 8.
12. Theurer, Dan. "How to Build a Maps Mash-up." (November 3, 2005). Available: <http://www.theurer.cc/blog/2005/11/03/how-to-build-a-maps-mash-up/>. Accessed: November 22, 2006.
13. Rosen, Zack. "Screencast: Drupal Mashup Machine." (April 5, 2006). Available: <http://zacker.org/screencast-drupal-mashup-machine>. Accessed: December 8, 2006.
14. Darlene Fichter's Home Page. Available: <http://library2.usask.ca/~fichter/>. Accessed: November 22, 2006.
15. Butler, Declan. "Mashups Mix Data into Global Service." *Nature* 439, no. 7072 (January 5, 2006): 6-7.
16. "About HEALTHmap." HEALTHmap: Global Disease Alert Map. Available: <http://healthmap.org/about.php>. Accessed: November 22, 2006.
17. "About Vimo." Vimo: Comparison Shopping for Health. Available: <http://www.vimo.com/html/about.php>. Accessed: November 22, 2006.
18. iSpecies.org–a species search engine. Available: <http://darwin.zoology.gla.ac.uk/~rpage/ispecies/>. Accessed: November 22, 2006.

19. Miller, Paul. "Personalisation Tool Scoops Library Services Mashup Prize." Research Information. (October/November 2006). Available: <http://www.research information.info/rioctnov06library.html>. Accessed: November 22, 2006.

20. blyberg.net. "Go-Go Google Gadget." Available: <http://www.blyberg.net/2006/08/18/go-go-google-gadget/>. Accessed: November 22, 2006.

21. OCLC. "About Ross Singer's Umlaut." Available: <http://www.oclc.org/research/announcements/features/umlaut-about.htm>. Accessed: November 22, 2006.

22. OUseful Info. "Amazon2OU Library Pivot Browsing." Available: <http://blogs.open.ac.uk/Maths/ajh59/007292.html>. Accessed: November 22, 2006.

23. Chilibot. "Chilibot User Manual." Available: <http://www.chilibot.net/manual.html>. Accessed: November 22, 2006.

doi:10.1300/J115v26S01_10

Index